Perspectives on Vision--III

Selected papers from the Northwest Congress

Compiled by Willard Bleything, O.D.

Edited by Paul A. Harris, O.D.

Optometric Extension Program Foundation

Copyright © 2010
Optometric Extension Program Foundation, Inc.

Printed in the United States

> Published by the Optometric Extension Program
> 1921 E. Carnegie Ave., Suite 3-L
> Santa Ana, CA 92705-5510

Managing editor: Sally Marshall Corngold
Cover design: Kathleen Patterson

Library of Congress Cataloging-in-Publication Data pending
Perspectives on Vision--III
ISBN 0-929780-29-0

****

Optometry is the health care profession specifically licensed by state law to rescribe lenses, optical devices and procedures to improve human vision. Optometry has advanced vision therapy as a unique treatment modality for the development and remediation of the visual process. Effective vision therapy requires extensive understanding of:
- the effects of lenses (including prisms, filters and occluders)
- the variety of responses to the changes produced by lenses
- the various physiological aspects of the visual process
- the pervasive nature of the visual process in human behavior

As a consequence, effective vision therapy requires the supervision, direction and active involvement of the optometrist.

****

Table of Contents

1971
Optometric Visual Training   1
J. Baxter Swartwout, OD

1971
The "Team Approach" Care of Child   111
    Vision Problems
Paul Dunn, MD

1972
A Pediatric Look at the Mal-adapting Child   142
Ray Wunderlich, MD

1979
Nutrition and Vision   178
Phillip H. Taylor, MD

1982
Vectographic Techniques for Binocular   199
    Refraction
Irving Borish, OD

PERSPECTIVES ON VISION III
Northwest Congress

FOREWORD

Paul Harris, OEP Vice President

The *Perspectives* series was conceived as a way to bring, to a larger audience, some of the more interesting and thought-provoking papers in the archives of the forums and symposia held under the auspices of the Optometric Extension Program Foundation (OEP). *Perspectives III* features the Northwest Congress which gave its speakers the opportunity to give extended presentations. Fortunately, these presentations were recorded and transcribed by Dr. Carol Croissant and are now part of our rich, recorded heritage.

Most of these presentations were only heard by the people who attended the Congress. They represent a distillation of years of clinical experience and frequently, the presentations represent hours of effort grappling with concepts that are central to developing an understanding of behavioral aspects of the visual process. These presentations illustrate the efforts to organize and express these concepts.

Dr. Willard Bleything graciously consented to review transcripts covering many years of the meeting. As editor, I take this opportunity to thank Dr. Bleything for his invaluable service in helping to select the papers in this and in *Perspectives IV*, which you will see soon, both of which come from this amazing meeting. Thanks to Dr. Bleything for his fine efforts on this volume and for all he has done, throughout his career, for his patients and for the development of behavioral vision care worldwide.

Additional thanks go to those who served as preliminary editors of these papers. This includes: Barry Cohen, Clint Hoxie, Elizabeth Jackson, Steve Nicholson, Margaret Ronis and Wayne Yorkgitis.

INTRODUCTION

NOTE: Because these are transcripts of oral presentations, reference citations are not formally done. This is not a refereed publication. In addition, in the editing changes from the direct transcription were made to help readability, but for the most part the style has been kept as a written form of the spoken text. No attempt was made to put this into formal writing form. Also note that few of these presentations have titles. We do not have the programs from these presentations. As a result we don't have a record of the titles they used at the time these were given.

The Presenters

1971
J. Baxter Swartwout, OD

Dr. Swartwout dedicated his life to serving his patients, the profession and the community. He served the OEP in many capacities over the years including President of the Board of Directors. He took many opportunities to share his knowledge with his colleagues and published a significant amount of material that was always extremely helpful and practical. This presentation is unique from his other writings in that he shares a depth of insights and the "why" as he developed his understandings in a clinical way. This piece is timeless. As I edited it I could hear the instructors of the OEP Clinical Curriculum saying many of the exact same things. I am grateful to Dr. Bleything for finding this marvelously insightful piece into Baxter's genius, so that others may benefit from his expert ability to make his thinking and his clinical insights explicit.

1971
Paul Dunn, MD

Dr. Paul Dunn was the pediatrician we wish each of us had in our community. He was not just open to new ideas and worked with optometry as an equal partner but he helped open up exchanges with optometrists to further the learning and knowledge base of both professions. In a way he functioned like a catalyst to bring about a significantly bigger change than one expects from any single person. His insights about movement and early childhood development are still very timely today. Perhaps sharing this section with pediatricians could help facilitate opening up new productive collegial dialogue.

1972
Ray Wunderlich, MD

Dr. Ray Wunderlich was a long time friend of optometry. Here he shares his perspectives on many of the things that we also address clinically. He greatly anticipated the attention deficit disorder (ADD) and related conditions epidemic, but from a different point of view. His background and strengths in neurology and functional development come across loud and clear. Here is another MD who really related well with optometry because he saw very similar aspects of human performance from similar perspectives. He saw the vast majority of the difficulties that children had as amenable to change through alterations of the environment. For him this included optometric vision therapy, lenses, nutrition and many other factors as well. So often the red flag of chronic earaches is a trigger for the child getting off of the road of normal development. Dr. Wunderlich shares his clinical insights as to what is going on when this happens. This information should help every health care provider have a better way to explain how something as innocuous as an earache could have strong ramifications.

1979
Phillip H. Taylor, MD

Dr. Phillip Taylor is another pediatrician whom each of us wishes we had access to in our practice area. In this presentation he shares a tremendous amount of insight into how nutrition affects the person, their visual development and many other factors of how a child learns, or doesn't learn, in the classroom. If every pediatrician knew now what Dr. Taylor knew back in 1979, we would not have had an epidemic of overuse of stimulants to treat ADD and its variants. This presentation is as timely now as it was in 1979. *In a few instances where a drug name or a supplement name has been changed, I have attempted to find current information and insert that into the text or into the footnotes.*

1982
Irving Borish, OD

Dr. Borish is an icon of the profession and is probably most famous for his marvelous and comprehensive reference book, *Clinical Refraction*. In this presentation he brings to the group his thoughts on, what was at that time, a new direction for the profession. Indeed he presaged a massive burst of activity in this area that now seems to have leveled off. He spoke about getting space and binocularity into the optometric examination and, in particular, using vectographic techniques to isolate what each eye sees but to also have it be as natural as possible. Many have used the "Borish Vectographic Card" in their examinations. Here he talks about this revolutionary new way to evaluate how a person uses their visual process.

Dr. J Baxter Swartwout Optometric Visual Training 1971

Lecture I

I guess you might say that my "bag" is visual training, children, learning, and optometry… and, really, that's what I'm going to be talking about. I'm going to talk about a point of view that I take with parents… because I think they also exercise some responsibility and control over the development of the child—the visual segment of it—the problems we deal with. Because of that parental involvement, if we can begin to arrange conditions in our office and then extend those conditions as much as possible to home, I think we've gained considerable control in organizing our training programs for the resolution of visual problems.

Now in doing this, about 12 years ago, I kind of "had it" one day when I received more than one call canceling the arrangements that had been made with the one parent to come in with the visual analysis with the child. I said, "Let's see if we can't stop this. This is a waste of time." I dream about those kids at night. Sometimes months after one of these canceled appointments, I'll wake up and be thinking, "I wonder what happened to them?" And maybe I never found out. I have minimized this sort of thing by requiring both parents to be present during the initial examination of a child. Now there are exceptions and the rule is broken but, in general, this is a pretty hard-and-fast rule. The appointment is made with this rule in mind, regardless of who the individual is. (I'm thinking in terms of other professionals.) I want those parents there if they want me to deal with a visual problem. I don't think I'm being high-handed in this. I'm simply trying to consider the limited amount of time that we have for examining. I know I have to examine a certain number of patients a year in order to develop the visual training program that I do have in the office. The more of these mismatches we have with people who cannot see my point of view at the outset, and who I've already spent an hour with, then the more I'm going to have to see to make up the difference.

So, perhaps I'm limiting a certain segment of the population at the very outset when they call the office to ask for an appointment for their child, when we say that both parents will come. Usually, the receptionist will say, "What will be a good day for your husband?" That's how the ice is broken, because 9 times out of 10, or more, it's the mother who calls. So, this is arranged right at the outset.

We also use a pre-examination questionnaire (that is a very short form) so that I can begin to have some insight prior to the time of seeing the child and the parents of what they consider to be the reason for the child being there. I've been asked by optometrists, "How can you do that? How can you require both parents there when the questionnaire would indicate that there's no learning problem?... that he is there because he has failed the nurse's test at school… which you could have found out without even the questionnaire?" And I say, "Well, for these parents, I also want them there because I find it very much easier to make my recommendations and have them followed through when both parents are there. For example, when it comes to any lens application, which may be a bifocal type, when the father is there to see the reason for this recommendation, if this is indeed the recommendation, I can expect better follow through. It also makes it a great deal easier to make some hygienic-types of recommendations (that we will see as we go through the examination), which we try to communicate for the father and the mother both to see the reasons for these recommendations, hoping for continuing some of the observations to the home."

So I have, then, that questionnaire to look at. Incidentally, my assistant usually goes over this and red-checks the items that would be of particular interest, as she deems it, and then I can review it very quickly by those red-checked items.

The day of the examination, the day that the child comes in, they are ushered into the examination area, where I usually leave them for just a couple of minutes to look around and get oriented to the place. Given that time to get acquainted, we can usually, pretty quickly, get involved with testing.

I begin by thanking the parents for the information that they've already given me, explaining that it has helped me to understand something of the nature of the difficulty so we can minimize the amount of time necessary to draw out these things. I will ask some specific questions. This is particularly true if the parents have used some language on the questionnaire that would indicate, in their words, "The child has a visual motor problem." or, "The child has a visual perceptual problem but no visual motor problem." I have seen things like this on these forms and you wonder where these parents get this kind of language and get these kinds of ideas. So, sometimes you find it has to do with their own background, which I'd like to know about if they have a background of language of this sort. To some degree, it's going to have an effect upon my own language with them. Or if this is language that has been parroted from someone else, I would like to know who has told them this, because this individual probably should get a report, and this comes out in the discussion later.

The first "test" we do in the examination is with the child seated at the school desk that we have right near the consultation desk, with the parents seated around it. One of the things I don't do (at this point) is to try to instruct the parents as to their behavior during the examination. I purposely am saying this at the outset because it's part of the plan I utilize in the examination. This kind of question has been brought up and sometimes I forget to describe it during the course of describing the test. So, by way of explanation, what we look for, are the parental reactions to the situations that we are going to introduce that are visually oriented. I want to see whether or not they become annoyed... or overly helpful... or whatever reactions that the test may engender in the parent. I want to see this... especially if this turns out to be a case that we're going to be working with them in visual rehabilitation. I want to know the kind of parent I'm going to be working with. Because the possibility is that some of the same attitude I see, and which I will mention it once I've observed it, I'll tell the parent, "This is very hard for you to sit there and observe things like this without trying to help him, or without getting upset about it. But what I'm interested in is his reaction to these test situations as I state them to him, not so much your reaction." That's what I tell the parent, though I really am very interested in both the patient and the parent.

So, back to the tests. We start out at the desk with paper and pencil tests. I find that I can get a lot of this information very quickly and

I may put a 12-year-old or 14-year-old on some of the simple paper and pencil tests, no less than a 6, 7, 8 or 9-year-old. There are some other reasons for it, too. But to start out, the first thing I do is a tactual haptic, which I guess would be a closer term for a haptic test or geometric form in which I have the child reach into a cloth bag and feel the shape. The shape of the first one he feels is actually a poker chip. The second one is a little square about the same relative size as the poker chip. The third one is a triangle and the fourth is a diamond. I have the child reach in the bag and feel the shape. Very specifically, reach in the bag and feel the shape. "Do not look at it. When you have felt it, make one like it on your paper. And to see a child 10 years of age reach in the bag, feel the shape and pull it out and look at it and then kind of look at you with a half grin—he knew what he did. But he's telling you something right here about his haptic understanding, very possibly. Now don't get me wrong. I'm not going to try to make an instant diagnosis on any of these findings and I'm not going to try to make a complete diagnosis on any one finding, anyway. But we try as we go along, whenever we have something that can be described meaningfully or related particularly to the information I already know, that the parents have told me that they know about the child, we will try to make a communications bridge immediately upon seeing a response. Not so much in a dogmatic statement, such as, "There's the problem. That's why he can't do this other thing that you've described here." …but more in terms of a question. "Do you notice a relationship between the way he performed on that test, or the way he handled himself here, to the way you described he handled himself in the classroom, or at ball play, or something of the sort?" We try to draw a bridge in this way without hitting them hard with dogmatic statements, but more or less with questions.

When the child has finished the four geometric forms on paper with pencil, I then use the Winter Haven copy forms. Now, at times, I get concerned that some people in a big group like this are going to get concerned that since this is what I say I use, this naturally must be the only, or the best, or "the" way to do it. And believe me, I don't believe this. I don't believe it for a minute. I simply describe the things I'm using… and the things I'm going to describe to you are very simple things… because I find that in making communication bridges between a very complex subject and the people involved, that simple communication sometimes is a little easier to deal with than complex testing situations, if I'm trying to make a bridge immediately.

So, I use the Winter Haven copy forms and I observe the child's performance, and frequently we will find the parents making comments here about the child's posture at the desk, about the way he holds the pencil, about the way he's organized the work on the paper, or something of this sort. And it's only then... when the parents begin to insert their own observations vocally or in other less obvious ways of body language... that we will then talk to the parents about trying to just sit there and observe, telling the parent that what we're really interested in is how the child understands the situation.

With some of the older children who we still use the Winter Haven copy forms with, some of the things that we can begin to communicate will be verified later on perhaps in the analytical examination, or perhaps in some of the ocular motor tests. But some of these performances would relate to the organization on the paper. A child at 8 or 9 years old who starts in the middle like a 5-year-old and then just scatters the things around... I mean, I'm interested in this kind of thing. I begin to wonder and just sort of look at the pre-history form (which usually I wouldn't have to because I've just kind of gone over it) to find what kind of math ability has been reported in this child? I have something to think about if I see him on the divided rectangle looking several times to produce the form, and yet the form, when you look at the finished product, looks quite decent. What kind of reading consistency does this child have? He may have a learning problem. He may have difficulties with reading. What kind of consistency does he have in word calling? I will frequently at this point, as early as this in the examination, ask the question of the parent, "Have you heard him read out loud lately?" Or, "Does he misread words that he has just read only a line or 2 above?" My own experience has been that many children who have to look several times to reproduce the form, despite a good reproduction in its final form on the paper, take a very small bite of visual information at any one time. And in the relentlessness of a reading task that is so on-going, in order to maintain continuity for comprehension, this child doesn't always have the time necessary to put all the pieces together to come up consistently with the same decoding of these visual symbols. At least my experience has indicated this kind of thing. And I ask the question very early in the examination, "Have you heard [the child read aloud]?"

Again, I don't try to tell the parents that he must necessarily misread or be inconsistent in his reading… because I've had a number who don't miscall words according to the parents' understanding of their child. Now this understanding may or may not be correct, but at least the parents haven't recognized it. Or maybe they haven't heard him read, so that we simply ask to find out.

I'm also very interested in postural aspects that we can see at the desk… aside from the parental reactions to these things… my own observation of them… the asymmetries that can be seen. As with one child the other day… and I'm sure it's not unusual for you to see it either… literally with a head tilt to the left and over to the arm and lying on the table. He couldn't have been more than 3 or 4 inches from the pencil tip with the right eye, and I'm quite confident that the left eye was not involved in the process as such on a teaming basis. Interestingly, the parents had already made note on the pre examination questionnaire (which they don't always in this particular regard) indicating that they thought the child many times did things so close that he could only use one eye. It's not often that we find this as a parental observation. But this was on it and the child demonstrated it at the desk without our having discussed it at this history, this very short history that we will take and maybe ask them further questions. That was an obvious enough thing that I didn't want to clue the child into this particular thing. I would rather see it. After seeing it, then we brought it up; then we asked about it; then we talked about it after we had observed it.

The other thing that, frankly, I'm very interested in is the grip… the intensity of that child's finger grasp of that pencil. The white-knuckled kind of intensity… I mean, I just cannot see any possibility of a child using himself really efficiently over periods of time under these conditions… not just in terms of the fingertip operation of the pencil, but in terms of the motor and the sensory operation of himself through time. I mean, any of us who have been under any kind of intensity in the shoulder or the neck or the hand or wrist area find ourselves stiffening up. We are certainly are not going to be able to use ourselves efficiently and fluidly and productively for long periods of time under these conditions. Any ball player will tell you if he's a little bit stressed or tense physically, he's not going to play a good game. Or if he's a little bit stressed or tense mentally, he's going to be a little bit stressed or tense physically and not going to play a good game. It's a two-way street, this mind and body, this organization of information processing and the resulting patterns that come from it. It is purposeful. It is an operation that is a closed circuit in this way, both sensory and motor, and the child who is doing this on paper and pencil, I see him as a child who is not using himself efficiently through time in a motor way… which is invariably going to affect the sensory areas as well. So, I may not say much about it at this moment. I may wait for other confirmation through other information that we should be able to get somewhere else in the visual examination.

Those two things we do at the child's desk. The desk is one of the American Seating Company desks with the 10/20 slope. After the deskwork, we will then say, "Let's go over to the big chair and take you for a ride." And he goes over to the big chair for the ride and the parent's kind of spread out a little bit so we have room.

The first thing we do would be visual acuity. I've said this before, that I could cry at the number of years I did visual acuities in a very cursory manner simply to get the visual acuity notated on the record chart… because I had been convinced as a student at Columbia that this was the first thing you did in case you flicked your finger in the child's eye and you found out that was an amblyopic eye afterwards, you wanted to have this measured before you'd stick your finger in the eye. Then you could always say, "Well, it wasn't my finger that did it. He had it before he came in." So, always record visual acuity first. But the point is it was done pretty much just to get a mark on the paper to protect myself. I was long since convinced that you couldn't write a prescription on the basis of visual acuity, so, really, that was about the only reason I did it.

In contrast to that, what I began to hear as I let myself observe rather than judge during the course of an examination… and began to observe more than just simply to get some figures to put down into the proper areas on the form… is all kinds of visual perceptual difficulties, visual spatial relationship problems, inconsistencies in information, stressed visual perceptual information. There are all kinds of possibilities in this thing.

For example, there is the child whom we see, not uncommonly, who when we've exposed the Snellen chart and say, "Do you see the chart across the room?" he says, "Yes." "Can you read the letters?" He says, "Yes." "Would you read the bottom line?" And he says, "D-A-O-6." That's the top line I have exposed. (At this time, incidentally, if we haven't already talked to the parents, I give them a quick look just to make sure that they're not about to jump into the thing, because I want to see what's going on here and I don't want them interfering with this. It's usually too good of a game.) I will say, "How about that line you read? Is that the bottom line?" And usually this child will come up, "Oh!" or something like that... surprised... momentarily surprised. I've had them then read two lines below to the 20/40 line... the "F-Z-B-D-4" line. And then I ask, "Is that the bottom line that you just read?" only to have another, "Oh!" and drop down to the 20/20 line.

Now, I ask myself something about this child's visual organization for spatial relationships. And I hear people in other disciplines describing their test for math readiness in the early grade levels before they're even handling figures, about these things, these spatial relationships of visual nature, the organization of math concepts. And I again check back to my previous test at the school desk on the paper and pencil and I see this lack of organization. And here's a child who has been in school for three or four years and he still is starting in the middle or he's starting at the bottom or he's starting on the right or he's just starting almost any old way, and he sometimes gets a form that's started out on the paper and then gets it half finished before he realizes he doesn't have enough room between that and the next form and then starts again. Or he changes the shape of the form to make it fit the space. Or, he just runs it right into the other form anyway, "What the heck." I can't help but wonder how this child handles other kinds of spatial relationships that would be necessary. From the visual standpoint... of being able to deal with one thing and then come up with something else that requires a differing point of view... when the child doesn't see the relationships at the physical, concrete level with things in my own hand and I can hear it confirmed on a visual test as simple as "Can you read the bottom line?" and I hear the top line read, I know that their visual difficulties are at the root of their learning problems. So then we would begin discussing with the parents right then and there the possible involvement of the visually-oriented problem or related problem to this child's academic difficulty.

Now, although all throughout the time I have with you I'll probably be talking very frequently about the academically disadvantaged child from our visual point of view, optometrically, I don't limit my practice or my visual training to this type of child. Nor do I limit my visual training to the child. We have some of the most beautiful academically disadvantaged adults in our visual training, because these same children do grow to adulthood, somehow, and some of them can manage to do pretty darn well despite their problems, despite their difficulties, but they make very wonderful training patients. So, I'm still going to be emphasizing, however, this orientation through the visually-disadvantaged, academically-disadvantaged child.

There is another thing that we will hear on the acuity test that I frankly found very fascinating, and I'm not sure that I can explain it to you any more than I can fully explain it to myself or parents. But, it's an interesting phenomenon, and, again, I'm sure that we've all heard it. I've heard it for many years before I began notating it or began thinking much about it. And that was on this particular A.O. chart we have that has the numbers on the far right; 6 at the end of the 20/60, 5, 4, 3, 2-5 at the 20/25 line, and 2 at the 20/20 line. That's on the right. As the child reads across the line... maybe this is one who has gone right to the bottom line when we say, "can you read the bottom line?"... he says, "Yes. E-V-O-T-Z-2."... but instead of "2", he says "E-V-O-T-Z --"...and he's read them very nicely up to that point, without the kind of slow, hesitating, uncertain response that is characteristic of another group of children. He'll read it right out... but then he stops. And you know, with some of these children, unless I really push it, unless I really crowd them, I get no response at all, by waiting or with a soft kind of question like, "Do you want to try it? What do you think it looks like?" No response at all. I go to the next thing. I say, "Try the line right above it." "A-P-E-O --," and he hesitates again when he comes to that 2 and the 5, and just as often as not, we'll get "Z-S." And we'll say, "How about the line right above?" "O-F-L-C-E." And the 4 at the end of the 20/40 frequently will be an "A". The 5 at the end of the 20/50 will, as often as not be a "5", and the 6 at the end of the 20/60, if we push it that far (and I normally don't, but I have). And I've gone up to the 20/70 line and I've heard the 7 called a "T". But what I do, not pushing it that far in most instances, I'll hear enough of this and I'll make an aside to the parents, "Perhaps you have an idea or a notion of what I'm trying to get at here, or what I'm looking for." And usually you'll get a nod, because they're looking at one another. Every time he says it's an "E" when it's a 3, what I do very quickly is to run that slide into the vertical column to expose the final right-hand column, all numbers from the 6 on down and ask the child to read that. Invariably, the child will say, "6-5-4-3-2." The 5, he'll sometimes hesitate, but as often as not get it. And even the 2 on the 20/20 line. And very quickly, without a word, I'll run it down to the little square and zip in the horizontal line, maybe at the 20/30 level, and about half of these kids will say, "O-F-L-C-E." The other half will now have picked up a relationship here and will say, "O-F-L-C-3" and you move back down to the 20/25, and they'll see the 2 and the 5, but a lot of them will not.

What is it we're dealing with here? It's helpful, clinically, at least, to look at and think about these things. This is one of the beauties of being a clinician. You are working with an individual with an individual problem. You already have a history. You have some understanding and some knowledge of how he's dealing with his other environments, utilizing the same visual system for information processing. It should be consistent in the other environments as it should be here, and we have perhaps, by observing closely, a chance to see some link between the way he understands his other visual environments by his responses to this very overtly simple kind of visual test.

And usually you will find, if you begin to question the parents at this point, they've seen this; they've heard this. The parents will begin to relate for you how he responds in other situations… where he begins to show inconsistencies in visual understanding and other environments that they see him in… or that insightful teachers have already described to them. Sure, he does his work and he's capable of doing a great deal of good work, but he is probably very inconsistent in doing it. This is one of the clues we would have with this child. Visually, perceptually, he is inconsistent. He may be able to center. He may be able to localize... but he's probably (if we begin to look at other relationships that we've likely already seen, maybe at the school desk)... he's probably a pretty tight little kid.

Can you see a relationship between tightness in this regard? Can you see that if I put on a visual test to identify these 'letters'... (because that's what he sees)... he starts at the left (he's learned this visually, at least) and he sees all these 'letters', and he's going to read letters. He's visually tight in this information processing type of situation of having to deal with little differences... little likes and differences all at the same time. And he's just not able to sort these things out that easily or that well and with that much assuredness. I ask sometimes, after the child has read the O-F-L-C-3 line and read the 3 as an E, I'll say, "Is that the way you make an E?" And he says, "No. That one's backwards." This is a thinking child but he's having difficulty shifting gears in a very simple dual symbol system that we've exposed for him. He's struggling to be able to deal from one point of view and then another point of view.

When we get involved in our visual training, we find that this is one of the children that we do have to reinforce continually for the parent that this ... this helping him to find a way in which he can keep himself flexibly alert in this visual area ... this is something we're interested in and something that we're going to have to work with.

I don't think we can do that effectively unless we also think in terms of the motor system. Not just ocular motor, but the general motor system... because as I indicated, these children generally speaking tend to be tight. (I'm going to have more to say about this kind of thing later.) These children are tight both in say, "Roll your shoulders around, the way you were before, like this, like that." "Wow," some of them say, and a line sometimes fades. I say, "Okay. Even with the shoulders, what you do there has some bearing upon this, of how you see and how efficiently you're going to be able to use those eyes and what you're going to do to yourself if something doesn't occur to change this kind of way you've been using yourself. Let's try one more. Keep the shoulders back, the chin back, and now can you slump." And you get another, "Wow," because there's another reduction in acuity.

Does this happen every single time you try it? No, it doesn't. In fact, I would advise you if you haven't done it, if you want to try some of these things with the kids, and begin to get some communication with them as well as with the parents, that you watch whether the child gives you a completely adverse response to this thing. Be aware of those children who's posture is like he still has a book in his hands, or the TV slouch or whatever you want to call it, when he does get up or sit up and he finds a way to do it, he's lost out there visually. He's no longer seeing as well. With enough of these children over the years, I have tried something and sometimes on these types of children who have visual acuity worsen with better posture, if they will do the experiment with you again and do this several times in the chair, thinking about getting the shoulders back, the head back and the back arched, and then slouch all the way again, and then back and forth, you'll get another kind of "Wow!" after maybe 3 or 4 or 5 times where they suddenly recognize they are seeing a reversal. Sometimes they don't say a word but you can read it on their faces and you can say it. "It's different now, isn't it? Its better when you sit up and it is worse when you hunch down."

What is perception… and where is it? How does it organize? What does it relate to? What is visual acuity but one little smidgen of this whole thing, of how I understand something? And we give credence to the notion that vision is motor as well as sensory… and that perception is an understanding… that it is something I put together through all kinds of experiences, not just at the sensory level but at the motor level… and that the gravitational and postural areas are involved in it. We say these things. We know these things. We can see these things and we can begin to communicate these things to the parents… where we can now, literally, begin to do visual training right at the outset from this examination… because any arranged conditions in that child's environment for improvement of the efficiency of this system for information processing is indeed visual training. It's one definition, at least, of it that I would go by.

Now we are also beginning to get the parents to recognize that we must be more involved and concerned than simply at the eyeball level of vision and seeing… that we have to involve more of the child as well as the parents in the training program… because the child is telling us that he needs a monitor; he needs somebody to help him; he needs somebody to observe so that they can maybe pat him on the shoulder or say a word here or there. "Remember what Dr. Swartwout showed you? Remember what you saw that day in the office?" When you see some of these children walk in the office a week later or a month later for the progress evaluation and see them sitting in the chair, and before I say anything to them about it at this point (I get some information first), but before I have a chance to say anything to the parent, "Gee, he seems to be sitting better. He's not all hunched down and slouched over." I'll have many a parent say, "I didn't say anything to him. I didn't tell him how to sit when he came in the office today. Did you notice the way he was sitting there today?" The parent is saying this. They're working together on something. We can see, as I have in one instance some years ago of two boys, brothers… one heard me and the other one didn't. At the annual reexamination, the guy who walked in the office differently, sat in the chair differently, and showed no increment in his myopia. (They were both nearsighted at this point, incidentally.) The other fellow who just didn't hear me, I didn't get to him. (I wish I did communicate to everybody - kids, parents, and what-have-you, but I can't.) This fellow… you could just see it. He was still in the posture that we had seen the year before and he had moved into myopia further. I don't know that this is the reason for it, but it helps to implement your own thinking when you can begin to see some of these things and see them through time with the kind of relationship that you would rather expect to find.

From the visual acuity test, I would next do a cover test. It's not too frequently that I communicate a heck of a lot with the cover test… but there are occasions and those are obvious enough, generally speaking, that I'm not going to go into them, very frankly… other than to make one additional comment. I do not try to impose little clinical value judgments that I may make of what appear to be small items on the parent. If it isn't obvious enough for them to see most of the time from across the room, I'm not going to pound this thing away or try to make a big case out of it. It may be very important to me… but if it is that important, there are going to be other things in the examination that I'll be able to point to later on to confirm this and to demonstrate this for the parents. I may then bring it back in and say, "I saw some signs or indications in some of the other tests that would have been a little difficult for you to see, but they also confirm the problem that we're seeing here now." So we'll move right on from the cover test, because I want to know what I'm working with behind that phoropter initially.

My next test in sequence would be the analytical. It is habitually my practice to do an analytical on anybody I can and I've been amazed at the age levels that I can move into and get findings on the analytical. Just what they all mean, I'm sure I don't know, really, except for this… It is a very sophisticated kind of test, any test we do behind the phoropter. Any time we put a disassociating prism before a child and say, "How many do you see?" we're asking him a rather sophisticated question that he has probably not had prior experience with. There is nowhere in his usual, normal, visual, living environments that he's had this kind of circumstance, and he can by no means reach out there to confirm this information by hand. And much of his visual data that he can rely upon, that he can work from with any degree of consistency, has been and can be confirmed by other motor or sensory information. But under these conditions, he cannot confirm these kinds of tests.

So… any child who responds to this testing, who will give me answers to these questions, is responding at a fairly sophisticated level of visual performance, in my opinion. Maybe I find nothing in the analytical that I can communicate to the parents. This does not mean I have found nothing to communicate to me. I may have the whole story right there. I should have. I should have a great piece of it. But I may not be able to communicate much to the parents other than I will say that he did rather well, or whatever, on this test that we have just completed, which is a very sophisticated level of visual performance.

However, there are a number of children who, on your first disassociation test will sit there as though they were dummies where they haven't been responding this way at all up to this point. Now, suddenly, you can't get responses… at least without pushing, without questioning, and without re-questioning. "How many do you see?" Or, you'll hear other responses that are mismatches in information processing that the parents can even hear. As the other day with a child (it has happened now twice within the past several weeks)... I will say, "Do you see the 2?" He said, "Yes." I said, "Where is the top one?" He said, "On the bottom." (laughter) I said, "All right." This could be, but I push it just a little bit further to get some further information. I can't recall specifically now. This is one of the problems of being a clinician, because I don't keep statistics up here and I don't keep in my own head findings on the different kids, other than isolated things that sometimes make a good illustration. I can't even remember this child's face or name but I remember that particular response.

But when I'm working with that particular child, I would almost be willing to bet... (I say "almost" because I don't bet. I lose usually.)... I would almost be willing to bet that I had corroborating information in that visual analysis that would have indicated other spatial relationships that this child has had trouble with that would have shown up maybe on visual acuity or maybe elsewhere. Whenever we hear this kind of mismatch in performance in response to the test situation, we can again draw a bridge first to prior tests that we have done... this one might have been related to the visual acuity test, or it might have been related to the paper and pencil test... and then to the observations, the knowledge that the parent already has of that child. So we're continually trying to bridge this gap of understanding to find out, "Just what is the problem? Just where does the visual system lay in this relationship of difficulty that they have brought in?" And what we very often will find is that it relates to difficulties that the child has had that they haven't told me about.

How many times have you, in using pre-examination questionnaires, for example, where questions about the child's academic level or standing, and so on... gotten a response of "No problem at all." And you get part way through this kind of evaluation and things begin to spill over. Then they begin to tell you about it. But they really didn't think it was any of your damn business in the first place, because they really didn't understand why they were coming to you, other than perhaps somebody had referred you to them as being good... for what I'm not sure... but good. So they come to you because they really don't know what to expect anyway from anybody else. Therefore, they're not going to give you too much information. I mean, you get this with adults sometimes. Not as often any more...

the cagey old fellow who you start asking a history and he just clams right up. He says, "You find out first and then I'll tell you." Fortunately, you don't run into too much of that. But I've heard it. And you get the feeling that you're dealing sometimes with some of these very close-to-the-chest parents. Either they don't want to identify or recognize some of the information you ask for… or they do think it's just not important. After all, you're going to make up glasses for them perhaps if he needs that sort of thing. But they don't identify this area with your work yet.

But do this kind of communicating. Even these parents can frequently, by the end of an hour, become very much oriented to the role of vision in information processing from the analytical. And, again, there are a number of things in the analytical that we can communicate sometimes other than phorias. One thing I would mention because, again, it runs against the training I had, is that when we disassociated, we were always taught to impress upon the patient (and now the parent sitting there) our understanding of exactly what we were doing when we said, "Now you see the top one on the right." "Yes." What I do now, I say, "Do you see the 2?" And if he does say, "Yes," I say, "Where is the top one?" And instead of getting, "On the right," you may get a good long hesitation, or we may get no response, or we may get left. And we say, "Which hand is that?" and he raises his right. In other words, with a very simple question on where this is, we can begin to get some further information about the laterality and directionality relationships of this child on this particular test. Because he's having difficulty in this very sophisticated type of situation where he can't get his hands to confirm what he's saying doesn't necessarily mean that because he says, "Left," and he raises his right hand, when you get that phoropter away and say, "Raise your right hand," that he's not going to raise his right hand. He may very well, but at least we know we have some confusion here, some inconsistency here in this area of relationship to the visual system.

Lecture II

We will move right along from the analytical to the eye movement test. The first one that I do, characteristically, is the near point of convergence. Largely, I do this first, because I find such an amount of pay dirt here for communicating to the parents. And again, much of the predictiveness of going to it is extrapolated from the analytical examination in the handling of these deductions. Much that I see here I see in the phorias. But it doesn't always relate one to one, either. What I look for is, first, the near point of convergence and how he handles himself in doing this, what kinds of intensities, what kind of frowning, what kind of tightness around the eyes and gritting of the teeth, or pulling away from the target as it nears him. Or release of one eye while he's still fighting with the other one to hold on. What kind of things we see.

And then I look for the recovery. Again, I don't know how many years went by before these very obvious things that can communicate so beautifully not only to the parent but to you as an optometrist I overlooked or just didn't bother with, or I just didn't see. If I did them, I didn't see them. At least I look back at my records and there's no notation about it in the records and I don't recall doing it. But the thing is, we see a child with a near point of convergence and they come in to 3 or 4 inches with a nice release, which I would much rather see than to have them just hang on to this thing, because I relate this kind of intensity to too many other potential problems for the future if we can't get him to get off before coming in too close. With the recovery there are some where I may—on the little stool I sit on—go back 3, 4, 5, 6 feet before he says, "Ah, it's one." And you can see that tiny flick, which indicates that this fellow hasn't been fooling. Usually it isn't that bad, but I have seen a number of instances where it has gone back that far before we got a recovery after a decent near point break. It's not uncommon to find the recovery at 12, 14, 15, or even 16 inches after a rather reasonable near point of recovery. But what kind of prediction can we begin to make for this youngster who's working in this—you can visualize this—such a fragile, visual, binocular area as this, where the break and the recovery is so close to where they do most of their near work? I don't think we have a youngster who's going to be able to sustain over long periods of time successfully. He may do it and this may be part of the problem, but I think we're going to find these other adversities of stresses that we will find where they begin to recognize fewer relationships in dealing with a task under these kinds of intensities. Where they just don't make the kind of broad perceptual, conceptual associations for the information they're dealing with. It's more goal oriented to get-it-done kind of thing, and they may get it done, but without a real good learning experience coming from having gotten it done. Because this, to me, is a very important part of what we can do when we establish a training program.

But first we must establish with the parent that what we're seeing here communicates perhaps a beginning reason why this child is working the way he is working. Or, avoiding working the way he is working. Because it can go either way depending upon the temperament of the individual, how much they expect of themselves and what kind of a self-concept they still have of themselves. So for the same response, optometrically, we may get an entirely broad range of responses on the part of the organism to the same task demand. But this is what we can begin to communicate. It doesn't always have to mean that because we see a good break and a poor recovery that he must therefore always perform in such-and-such a way. There may be a very wide range of possibilities for this child's performance with this kind of observation. Clinically, this is where we can begin to communicate because that's all we can do with that parent—communicate what we see and relate it to what they have already seen in the child's performance.

It's not just near point of convergence but near point of convergence and recovery. We see the obvious poor near point of convergence of 12 and 14 and 16 inches with a child who still is not reporting diplopia, a child who has never told anybody that he sees double, and indeed may never have seen double under his usual conditions. Some of the parents will begin to pick a thing like this up as you begin to point this out as a possible problem. That here he is with a break where they can see the eye flip out at maybe 16 inches and he's reading at 12 inches and he's never reported seeing double. What do we do? I repeat the test with the near point target held against a reading card with the print vertical. I mean, I'm not asking him to read even, just the near point card as a greater ground around the figure and move it in. Many times you will find the same child who broke on the near point bell or ball or whatever you use, who broke at 16 in. come in to a much better, more usual, normal kind of near point of convergence if he has more ground around the figure you're using for the test object.

But qualitatively, we've still learned something, that this child is having difficulty with his Centering mechanism. And very likely, if he's having difficulty with Centering, he's going to have trouble with localization, with knowing where things are spatially. In my own thinking, this is where our understanding for Centering comes from. It is knowing where the thing is so that I can center upon it. If I have to have a bigger bite of information of the space relationships in order to be able to deal with this center, I don't see this child as being an effective, academic organism—not in our kind of culture. There's too much high intensity placed on Centering.

The next test I do would be the near-far fixation. One thing I have learned is not to try to play Russian roulette with these things. What I mean is, just because I see good performance on near point of convergence and recovery I should not skip testing near-far fixations. I've seen too many kids who can't do a good near-far fixation after showing mc a good near point of convergence and recovery. I've seen the other way around, too. You can think about the reasons, optometrically and physiologically and spatial relationship-wise yourself. But the point I would make here is that we can make a point again in communication to the parents with information that they've already told us that they know about the child. Continually, all the way through it, we will begin to relate these things to things that we see in the history, things that they've done—perhaps copying from board to desk or difficulty in completing assignments. Many times when I ask, "Have the teachers told you that he has difficulty perhaps in completing assignments that are written on the chalkboard, or writing, or copying work from board to desk?" Frequently the parents will say, "Not only that but even in transferring information from his workbook to paper." I've missed my bet because I haven't even done a saccadic fixation with the child yet. They're already jumping, they're already making a relationship because this is a type of saccadic too, only it's on the Z axis saccadic in this direction, rather than the usual testing direction of right and left.

The next thing I do is not a saccadic but a pursuit. This we do both binocularly and monocularly. I'll not tell you about my tears over this, but we will, many times, be able to further our communication with the parent, or maybe for the first time in the testing make our communication break with the parent on the differential that we will see in pursuits between the right and left eyes. What I normally do is to use information that Spache[1] made available back there in 1944, that some testing and observing that they were doing at the University of Florida in their reading at that point related to eye movement patterns. That many of the children who were being referred to them for reading help at the University were found by Spache and his associates to exhibit poor eye movement ability on pursuits. What they did further was to test these children monocularly as well as binocularly. In many of them, they found a differential that they as educators were able to observe and note. What they did, they set up a study of reading level testing with these children who met this particular criteria of a differential between right and left eye on pursuit testing and found that with these children, they would measure differences in reading level on graded material between right and left eye that would be as much as a year's difference in reading ability, or more in some instances. They also tested grade level with the binocular performance.

What they found with the binocular testing, which is I think of particular interest to us as optometrists, was that the reading level binocularly was never as good as the reading level achieved by the better of the two eyes alone. So if we have a child who is not working up to potential and who has difficulties in his work in school with his reading and so on, think how much more difficult this would be for this kind of child if we know that a binocular problem has this kind of depressant effect upon reading level. He is not even that much of a reader yet, he's just building the system for reading at this point, perhaps, so that he's that much more handicapped. If he's already moved through the learning-to-read stage and is in the high level, maybe this is something we would see then as a secondary problem that is now going to hamper his utilization of this ability that he has learned in reading. We have some clues to this. We have some clues as clinicians, again, by question. Did the child start out with a problem, for example, with his reading? Did he start out at a disadvantage academically initially, or is this something that has come about in the past year or two, or in 3rd grade or 4th grade?

With some also, the analytical would help us to clue in on this particular child; where he stands developmentally. Whether it's a

---

1. *George Spache – Inventor of the* **Spache Readability Formula** *which is readability test for writing in English. It works best on texts that are for children up to fourth grade.*

stress induced kind of problem or something more developmentally oriented, that he already owned before he ever set foot in the school, versus the problem that has been induced by the containment, the constraint, or the intensities that were perhaps induced on a not too stable development of vision. With this we can get into a lot of communication on these kinds of differences that have somehow apparently been meaningful to the parents that I see. I don't think that the parents I see are that different from the parents any of you would see.

The final—usually final test that we do in the chair at this point is a saccadic. The saccadic movement is at this point of very little value in communicating with parents at the level of eye movement ability, as far as I'm concerned. The undershooting, overshooting, various things of this sort that I can see, generally speaking, are slight enough that it becomes one of those things that's hard to communicate to the parent. As a result, for a long time, I didn't use this, until I realized I had another test here in a saccadic that was perhaps even more vital because I had so many other ocular motor tests that I could do anyway. In particular was the relationship between the auditory command that I'm giving the child and the visual response that he produces. The mismatches that we see there have been sometimes kind of scary, to the point where one child, showed a blepharospasm that I have never seen the likes of, at a time when he recognized that he was no longer looking where he was hearing was supposed to be looking at. I think he tried to do something about it and couldn't and he just went into a spasm. It was a real scary moment. It hurt.

But we do see—not usually that degree of reaction to this, but the child who even on a rhythmic presentation of orange-white, orange-white, begins to anticipate and begins to get to the orange before I have said it. And by the time I then say "orange," he's back to white and he now picks up the rhythm again and he's mismatched and doesn't hear the mismatch between what he's listening to and what he's seeing. He's looking at the white when I say "orange" and the orange when I say "white," and he goes on in blissful ignorance of this mismatch. This is a different child from the one who recognizes it immediately and makes the match again. I point this out to the parent because I don't stop there with this youngster, or with any of these. I will then do it without a clear rhythm. I tell them, "I'm going to goof it up this time. You're really going to have to listen!" I'll say, "Now listen carefully." And I'll do it out of any discernable rhythm. Some of them just can't handle this at all. Again, others recognize the mismatch and make great effort to try to be at the right place at the right time. But as I tell the parents afterwards, and the child too, I say, "You can fool anybody on this kind of thing. That isn't what I'm trying to do!" And if they have been able to monitor and wind up eventually on the right color when I have finished, I compliment them on this. I say, "You did know where to wind up." This is different from the child who winds up because I've finished talking and he's in the wrong place and doesn't recognize it. Again, we look for these matches and mismatches.

We can begin to get a little bit of understanding of how this child puts his auditory and his visual space together. The youngster who gives me trouble on this, where we can demonstrate it for the parent, I will often ask the parents if they have had complaints from the teacher that he doesn't pay attention, that he doesn't hear when he's spoken to. There are other ways and other kinds of problems that this kind of thing will work into, but at this point this kind of child usually is one who has had this kind of complaint registered against him. In fact, the parents will usually indicate to you that, yes, they had trouble too getting him to take auditory information and deal with it. But you see, the classroom is not just a visual world, it's a visual and an auditory and an everything-else kind of world. I often wonder—in fact, I do ask the parents—I often wonder how this child responds to audio-visual aids. How does he handle this kind of a situation? What kind of an aid is it for him, when he can't monitor the mismatches between where he's looking and what he's hearing? This child, the parents will tell you—usually, if they have been looking into his difficulty and they've been trying to fight the system to find out and get some help for him, that he has one heck of a time, he dreads audio-visual aids. He can't handle these things; it's too much for him. He can't deal with the projector sound there, the teacher's voice there, or the speakers there and the screen up there and his papers on his desk that he's supposed to put together in one piece. He can't put these together in one piece. He may have enough trouble just putting the visual aspects of it together such as shifting from near to far and back again. Now add another dimension at an auditory visual level to put together. We have some very interesting communicating bridges that we can make on a saccadic fixation as we begin to see these mismatches and misfires and lack of monitoring within the system.

There are other tests that I will do, usually led into it by the child, or perhaps to nail down additional communication, or for information for myself. But normally at this point in most of these children, I have gathered enough information to confirm for me that I have a visual problem that I would like to work with and I've been able to communicate to the parent that I know something about the problem that they begin to recognize that what they're seeing optometrically matches what they know about their child, and what they know school-wise about this child, because they have sat in classrooms, too. They know what it's about.

We would then go to the desk. If there are lenses involved—and you know, I completely forgot one of the very important things that I do in the examination. I would repeat any of these patterns we see difficulty with the lenses that were indicated by the analytical. Or if no indication for lenses there, by some kind of a probe lens. I might have gotten that information, if not from the analytical, from some of the other more sophisticated retinoscopic tests—the bell, or book or something of the sort. But I will repeat this because I will find a group of these children who will respond immediately to a low-powered plus lens and no longer show the lack of recovery in the near point of convergence. Or who will show a near point of convergence that is now adequate where they didn't show it before. Or where the pursuits will begin to smooth out where they were ragged and erratic before. Or where they can listen to me now on the saccadic. I want to know this and I want the parents to know this, because I know I can do something if they respond this way, and I can talk to the parents accordingly.

On the other hand, if the child doesn't respond favorably to these lenses, this is just as important for me and for those parents to know about. I may still want to use lenses and I may still have enough evidence that the lenses are going to protect what fragile skills he still owns at least, while we hopefully can help him to build some new ones in. But I can't expect to put lenses on him and have an immediate reaction, an immediate response. With some of the children whose motor systems may also work out nicely, I may not still be able to expect an immediate response. Suppose he has a problem with visual-verbal matching or suppose he hasn't really learned how to crack the code of our culture, reading in our language; so he hasn't been able to make this kind of a match. No matter how much I do with the motor system and the visual consistency of his circuiting of visual information, unless he's been able to learn how to crack the code, it's still not necessarily going to help him that much immediately with reading. So there are other possibilities in these things, and I think this is where we sometimes confuse ourselves as clinicians. When we see one good thing, we immediately expect another good thing to come from it. Fortunately, many times this is exactly what does happen, but if we are working from a base in strength and knowledge of our own information, we can make a better prediction as to what's going to happen with the use of the appropriate lens. When we finish the examination, I point out to the parents, "I do want to use lenses with your child." If I saw it and they saw it, I remind them of what we saw.

I point out to them that in spite of the fact that things look much better with those lenses on, the lenses can go just so far. They arrange some conditions out here in this environment but they do not necessarily change him inside. He's going to be able to use what he owns a little bit better but through visual training, we can help him establish more sound, better visual organization with which to meet these kinds of heavy demands. So that we would want to do the training to help develop the skills he owns inside and use the lenses to improve the efficiency that he's able to deal with in using the skills that he now owns. They will serve another function as we get involved in training in protecting these fragile new skills from the intensities of the classroom. We would want lenses and training, perhaps. But this is how we try to communicate the difference so we don't get the kind of unfortunate confusion that is very easy for a parent to assume, that the lenses straightened it out and the lenses are going to do the whole thing. You've seen enough of these instances where the lens do help a great deal, but in another 6 months, or another year or 2 years, you'll find that the case has deteriorated still further and the intensity of the problem is now greater. But they may still be using those lenses for effective goal-seeking; getting things done, but they're losing ground in terms of the depth and the breadth of the learning experience that we could have helped them with the lenses and the training.

At this point, if the parents decide that they think they'd like to go ahead with this visual training, I usually ask them to think about it and call me back. Lenses are going to be involved. It's going to take a week to get them from the laboratory and they can tell me about it when they come in for that. I want them to think about it. Again, I love training, I love the results of training but I hate to work with somebody who really doesn't want to work. I don't want to work with somebody that I'm going to have to prod constantly or push. When I was younger, more flexible and more saintly, I could work with them like that. But it's too hard. It's the hardest work I do, in planning and programming and evaluating these cases. I work very hard at it and I don't want disappointments. I don't want to spend a lot of time getting something organized only to find somebody changed their mind a week later because they didn't have at least a week to think about it. I'd rather have them pull out right then. So we ask them to think about it.

If they think about it and they want to go ahead with it, we then schedule what we call pre-training tests. These tests are done by one of my assistants. I'm going to spend what time is left describing some of these tests. I'll give you the list of them, even the ones I don't describe or spend any time on. I'll at least point out to you which tests they are. On this worksheet that we work from, it's simply a list of the activities that the assistant is going to do with the child. The form has three columns for three different test series that we might do—the 2nd one at the last training visit, for example, and a 3rd one for some other time. So we have these—it isn't a profile, it's simply a statement of the general condition under these test situations.

The first one is the Keystone Visual Skills. The Keystone plays a peculiar and a particular role in my diagnosis of a visual problem, because some of these children who aren't working up to potential or are, as I recall some of them, who are even in accelerated programs but working with great intensities, with perhaps considerable amount of symptoms and considerable amount of unhappiness, uneasiness about the role they're playing in this academically something-or-other environment that they produce in these accelerated programs.

I will frequently find that these children do not give me good demonstrations to communicate with the parents on these other tests that I have described to you so far. The analytical will tell me the story, but on these other tests, I don't see it—to communicate. I will, at the end of the routine things I've told you about, then go over to the other area of the training room and do a Keystone Visual Skills. Because what we often find, that we can begin to communicate to the parents, is suppression.

I remember reading that you shouldn't talk suppression to parents; you can't communicate with suppression. I think we can if we have a case that we're relating to; if we know something about this individual and how he's performing. If I find that this academically talented child who is in an accelerated program and unhappy in the situation, the Keystone test shows me a lot of inconsistency in the symmetry of his information processing at a visual level, I'm interested in it. Because one of the values I can point out to that youngster, who's usually an intelligent kid, and to the parents is that one of the great values that we have in binocularity is this simultaneity and this confirmatory aspect of information processing; that we have two circuits gathering this identical data, largely, to match within our system on a confirmatory note. What we're hearing here in his own words, in his own description of it, are mismatches of this information, inconsistencies in this information. I ask these kids, these talented youngsters, "How about your reading? Do you find yourself having to sit down when you read and re-read and re-read to be sure you get the information?" This is what they're doing. They are just grinding their gears down to a nub. They work so hard to get what they get, to produce those marks that they're still maintaining, to the point that the school will not take them out of their accelerated programs because they're still doing good work in that accelerated program. But they're paying for it inside.

With this kind of inconsistency in information processing, which I consider to be a type of asymmetry as much as this kind of thing is in a physical sense of the word, it's at a sensory level but it's an asymmetry in information processing, and this is how we communicate it to the parents. Then maybe if we can begin to get at this kind of thing so he can be more reliable and more consistent in this processing, with better matches in this processing, then perhaps we can do something to help him reduce the intensity with which he uses himself. We do. I love to work with these kids, because they'll respond very quickly. I've never yet seen one of them be removed from the accelerated program once we got them in training or even question whether or not they belonged in the accelerated program. And many of these children, the parents will tell you, have questioned the parents, "Do you really think I'm smart enough for the accelerated program? I don't really want to be in the accelerated program." They stop questioning this with the visual training and the consistency.

This is one of the uses we put the Keystone to. There are a number of ways you can communicate the problems to the parents. The second thing on our list for the assistants if I haven't done it in the initial examination is Harmon Circles. I would say that perhaps 3/4 of the time that I take the time to do the Keystone on the child, I will further take the time to do Harmon Circles with this child, because I see this kind of asymmetry in the sensory area that we call suppression in a very similar light to the kind of asymmetry that we would see in the motor area. That's why we go to something in the motor area and I look for asymmetries there, and you'll find them.

The motor system works off the sensory system. The motor system needs information to deal from. The binocular visual system is organized around the midline and so are the arms. It may be in this organizing of information around midline that he's having trouble with and it may not just be here at the visual level. I may not have seen it at the eye movement level visually but if we think of this kind of a movement as an information processing match also, we may still see it in a hand movement system where we ask the child, especially when we get to the point and now make them both go to the right," and he blithely goes right with the right and left with the left. You ask him if he is going to the right with both, sometimes monitoring and sometimes not. Or we then ask him, because again parents are alert to these things. Supposing the left hand is all wobbly and just miserable and this is all they see. We will tell the child, "Put your right hand down and just make the circles to the right and now to the left and now to the right." He has no problem organizing these movements with that left hand. Now we ask him to do it with the right hand, and he has no problem organizing these movements with the right hand. We say, "Now put them together and make them both go to the right." He goes into the same kind of crazy action, drop-out performance of the left hand.

What we point out to the parents is that he's having trouble putting information together, organizing teamed movement patterns that have to be based upon information that must cross midline. I relate it to the things that we saw on the suppressions and I point out that this is why I came to do this test. Because in our experience, we find that we can't assume that because he's having this problem at the visual level that this is where the whole problem is. That these problems generally tend to move through the whole organism, move through the whole system. Not always, not entirely. He may be able to relate at the leg level and not at the arm level or vice versa, but in general we will find on the Harmon Circles some confirmation of this sort of thing.

The next two activities are rotations and fixations. The fixation here is saccadic. I've already done this but we're going to do it again. We're going to do it differently. We're going to do it standing this time, and secondly, we're going to do it standing on a balance board. I have many records of youngsters who have shown me decent pursuits and saccades in the examination chair who fall apart when the thing is repeated standing up. Many more fall apart when they're asked to stand on the balance board. It's as though they cannot deal with the gravitational and postural world and the visual world—the world of movement, the world of muscle—without support in the chair. But to get the movement, the organization, the awareness of the gravitational reflexes under control, they must cut out. They have to withdraw, they must pull in somehow to organize these things and deal with it. Others will continue—they are dogged and they will continue on the eye movement activity at the expense of their postural and gravitational world. They're different children with similar problems of relating the visual gravitational worlds. There are so many interesting things that we will see about these youngsters, but again it's obvious the kind of communication you can begin to point out to the parents, so let me move right along.

The next three tests that we will do have to do with laterality and directionality. The first one, very simply—we refer to it on our list as laterality. What the assistants do is to ask the child questions about their own rights and lefts. The second one, directionality, we very simply ask him questions about our rights and lefts in different ways. He may be asked to touch, he may be asked to name, he may be asked to locate, for example, which ear did I touch, which hand did I use? We ask him different ways to express his level of understanding of this transformation of rights and lefts on the human body as they face one another.

The third test that we do is what we call pegboard. This has been described in the literature, developed at the Optometric Center in New York. Mickey Weinstein has discussed it. This is where the pegboard is used and the simple forms of. These are produced one at a time by the assistant. The child, not seeing her placement of them or the mechanics of her placement of them, but simply the exposure of the thing, is asked to make one like it. With youngsters who may be able to come up with answers of rights and lefts, even come up with answers to which hand is this of mine, which ear did I touch, and so on, but listen to them. Listen to the quality of this response. Listen for their hesitation. I read constantly the assistant's notes on this—hesitation, he must think it out, he sub-vocalizes it, he talks it out. All kinds of processing of this usually considered very simple thing of, which is your right hand or which is my right hand? These youngsters who must do this kind of processing will frequently produce the whole pattern reversed. You get flip-flops on this thing when they get their hands involved in it. Yet at a communication level verbally, they can describe rights and lefts, but they don't always see these reversals if they're not handling the relationships well. Or the other kids will get the pattern very accurately, but the notation by the assistant is, *used his fingers to count the holes to place the pegs.* There are all kinds of ways of getting the information out so that the goal is attained. These kids are trained to approach goals, to get work done, to get things turned in, and to get it done now. They're trained to approach goals, but they don't always understand the processes that they used to approach those goals. This is one of the things we'll work with the parents and the youngster in the training that we'll be discussing further on.

The next one we will do is the Van Orden Star. This characteristically has a very unique place because I would say that in better than 90 percent of the cases, it must run close to 100% of the cases, we will utilize this on the very last visit and do another Van Orden Star, and be able to point out something to those parents, that this child is now dealing from a different point of view binocularly. That there is either greater symmetry in the system, there is better centering in the system, there is a better eye-hand relationship that can be observed, there is something in this child's organization that is now different in his seeing ability. The value of this actually relates to the way I program the training and how we handle this. This is not part of what we'll be doing but we'll get involved in some of this sort of programming. But we utilize this so that the parents can recognize why I want that child now to repeat the home activities that they've been doing for 3 months, one week's segment at a time, and put it aside. The 2nd week another group of activities and then put them aside, and so on.

Now it's three months later. Go back to that first week's activities that he hasn't done for three months and redo it whether they look good, bad or indifferent, redo it, because this child doesn't see things the way he saw them before. He understands things from a different point of view. Even though it may look good now and look good the 1st week, he is seeing it differently inside. He understands it differently there, and this is where it counts. I point out to them that maybe it's only that he can now listen while he's doing the thing, but that's important. So we can use the same activities in a refining aspect than for the next several months or however long we program the thing. The Van Orden Star very frequently is the thing we can use to nail this down. The parents can hold it in their hand, they can look at the thing and they say, "Yes, he sees differently now. He understands something different now. I see what you mean. We won't just start dropping things out because it looked good the first time we did it three months ago."

The next two activities are gross motor activities. This time we work at the leg level. The Harmon Circles gave us some information of symmetry and organization at the arm level and now we'll have the child hop, we'll have him skip. Since these can be soft neurological signs to indicate to the pediatric neurologist possibilities of difficulty that he may or may not be able to confirm by other more sophisticated tests, he will still rate these as soft neurological signs if some of the motor acts can't be performed. I would like to know this, too, for my own reasons of organization around midline. Because I think we have an opportunity in our remedial profession to do something about some of these signs that other disciplines may relate to as a sign of other problems. At least that's been our experience that many times will change if we begin working with them. As a matter of fact, one of the children that we were working with about two years ago, who was still under the care of the institute for the development of human potential in Philadelphia and had been going back for some testing visits periodically, on a visit during the course of the training-we had been involved with the child maybe 1¼ months to 2 months when their appointment time came up. The mother asked if they should go back and I said, "Of course, any further information we can get is that much more, that much better." So they went back and when they came the next time, the first thing she said was, Dr. Swartwout, every time we've gone down there, the first thing they've asked Bobby to do is skip and he's never been able to skip." She said, "This time he skipped." I hadn't even gotten involved with skipping We have an activity sheet for it but I hadn't even assigned it. We hadn't even discussed it, but we had been working with eye movement prediction, visual prediction of hand, of eye, rhythm, listening, and monitoring his operations. He put the pieces together himself. They were all there apparently. He hadn't been skipping at home. The man said "Skip," and now he skipped where for the past two years he had not skipped. It was Kephart who said that the marbles are all there but he can't find them fast enough. Or maybe he just can't put them together in the appropriate way at this particular time.

The next four tests that we do are right out of the book of Abe Kirschner from Montreal. I think Abe has been at this meeting and he may have described this. One is visual count. This is his term for it. In visual count, the child is asked to count a series of dots on an 8½ x 11 piece of white cardboard. They're kind of organized in a random sort of circular way, but random. We have one card set that will have something from, anywhere from 7 to 11 dots on it. These dots are maybe 1/8 of an inch in diameter in India ink. And we have another set of cards that will have 20 or more dots on it. And we use it in two ways. We will say, "Would you please count the dots on this card, but do not count out loud, just count the dots." He comes up with a number. We notate it. If there were 21 dots on the card and he says 25, we notate it 21/25. We know which card we've used. If we want to retest, we can use one of the others. We then ask him—we pull out another card which has another series of dots on it and we say, "This time I want you to count them again but I want you to count out loud and touch the dots as you count them." Thinking in terms of reinforcement, of having the feedback from tactile and auditory, from speech that this might be easier—it is not always easier. In some instances it is easier, but this is what we want to find out. We find in some instances the only way the child can be reliable on things like is to get his hands on it. We find other children, once they get their hands on it, they can't deal with it. At a meeting, one that started this whole series off this fall at the New York State Congress, there was an educator in the room at a workshop we did and she was talking afterwards about a child who, on parquetry blocks, could verbally describe the placement of blocks in fairly complex arrangements that would verbally match the pattern that had been drawn or presented. But if the child was asked to do this with his hands without saying anything and match, he couldn't match or create patterns to match other patterns. But he could describe it. She said, "What is this?" I thought about it and I said, "Is he reading?" "Yes, he's reading. He's doing pretty well." I said, "I'd watch this." He was a young child, 1st or 2nd grade, I don't recall. I said that I'd watch him. This child is going to be wearing some pretty thick lenses before this is over." She said, "He already is." He's so highly visual with none of the really support areas to help to confirm, to monitor, to match with that he's all here. We've seen this with some of the cerebral palsy (CP) kids where they have mental intellectual potential that they have developed—invariably these kids will develop refractive conditions of rather high amounts. But that's another thing. But we do look for these differentials of whether or not they get support or is it deterioration in performance that we see when we bring in these other sensory areas.

The second of these four Kirschner tests that we use is auditory count. Again this is very simple. The child is asked to turn his back to the assistant and she simply takes a pen and taps a hard surface with the pen, rhythmically and asks him to count this. Again we stick in the same sequencing categories of around 10 and around 20, depending upon the age and ability of the child. The second way that we do this is out of rhythm and we ask him to count the number of taps this way. Again we notate it the same way. If the assistant tapped the table 21 times and he comes up with 21, we write 21/21 or 21 over whatever the count was that the child gave. But it gives us some information of the auditory processing sequencing in time, rhythmically and out of rhythm. This may relate poor performance on this to notations I have already made in the initial examination on his performance with the saccadic. It may relate to the information that we've already developed to communicate with the parent in terms of his ability to deal with audio visual aids at school, or what-have-you. But we look for more of this kind of communicating information at this time as well as additional information that we can now begin to do something about. Because when we find these kinds of problems, we can develop activities to help him to begin to monitor and process and deal with time, space and the visual area. Because this is how we do it, we tie it into the visual area, we tie it into a visual sequence from an auditory input and vice versa.

The same can be said of the next activity on the Kirschner test, which we call tactile count, where the child again is asked to turn his back to the assistant. She takes her pen and taps him on the shoulder, out of rhythm this time. We haven't bothered to do this rhythmically but we do it out of rhythm. Again, the same kind of sequencing the same number groupings of about 20 or about 10. And to see the number of children who can't tell you how many times they were touched, who will stop you in mid-test and say, "Wait a minute, would you start again?" Which we will do, but these things are all notated. It's a matter of efficiency then. He may come up with the right answer but it's a matter of efficiency then, too. If he doesn't understand what's happening on him, on his own skin at the periphery of his own space world, I don't think it's too far a stretch of the imagination to begin to think that he may have some difficulties in organizing time-space relationships and occurrences and sequences and other things in this external world, if he can't deal with the home base here.

We want to know, is this the kind of child we're working with? When we find these youngsters who can't understand what's happening on them, to them, this may very well be something of a longer element in terms of dealing with the problem. If he has problems with the next one, of the last of these Kirschner tests that we use, then he's just a little bit further down the scale. He is now given the pen or the hard object to tap the table 20 times or 21 times or 10. And he taps the table. It's counted by the assistant, the parents also. To see some of these children start out like this, and after maybe 25 or 30 times on the table, look up at you almost with eyes pleading, like they wanted to say, "Could I stop now? I don't know where I am or what I've done. I haven't been able to monitor my own operations. I really have lost track here. I know I'm doing what you said but time and space I'm lost in and I just don't know what I've done."

We've learned to do this in a second way. Incidentally, the way Abe Kirschner has described it is this way. There are no particular instructions visually. We've found a number of children who, having difficulty doing this, if we say, "Now close your eyes and tap the table 20 times, they can do it And we've seen others who will have trouble doing it with their eyes closed but can do it with their eyes open. So, again, we see a little differential between how they do these things. At least we have some kind of a clue relating the visual world with this kind of processing and monitoring of time-space in their own movement, their own processing.

The last test that we have used consistently over a long period of time is the tachistoscope where we want to get a digit span at a hundredth of a second. We use the tachistoscope throughout the training program but I do not go to digits normally in the first 2½ to 3 months with the child, except on the retest at the end of 2½ to 3 months. We will consistently use the Lyons and Lyons series, the A, the X and the P series. Sometimes we will get to some of the domino series, too. Now if the child can begin to deal with these kinds of spatial relationships, if we go back to our testing on digits again and we will begin to find an increment in the digit test. And we usually do. And more than that, we will usually find more or greater symmetry because we do the tach test monocularly. We'll find all the way from zero on one eye to 3 or 4, or 5 with the other eye, to smaller differentials. Where at the end of 2½ to 3 months

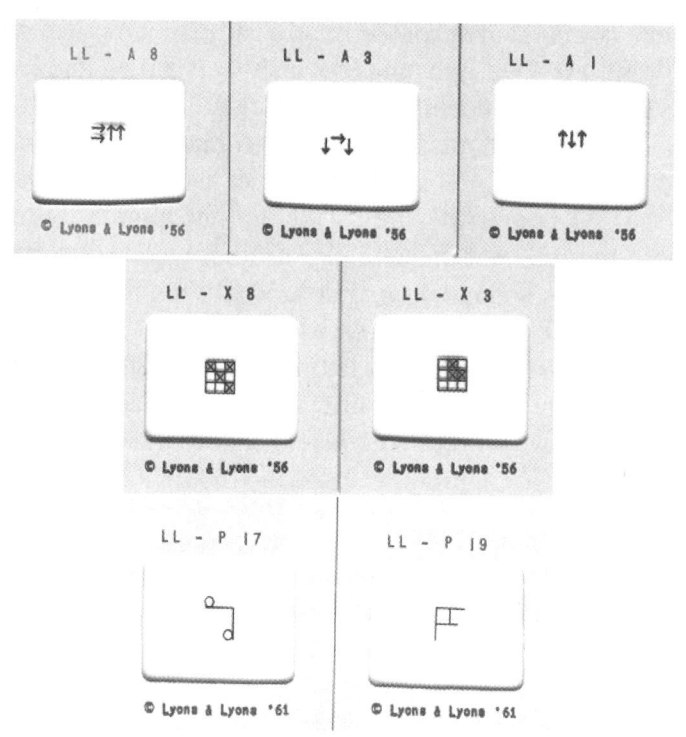

Figure 1. The above are samples from the Lyons and Lyons series of tachistoscopic slide series as mentioned in the text. The series of slides is currently being added to Vision-Builder ™ that includes a tachistoscope function that can be used in either direct view on a computer screen or projected on a marker board, chalk board or screen using a data projector connected to a Windows based computer. VisionBuilder ™ is available from OEP.

again, we begin to see, even in the zero to 4 or 5 differentials, greater symmetry where the other eye begins to be able to respond in this kind of timed information processing relationship.

There are two other tests that we do. One of them is alphabet array. This has been described in some of the Eastern Seaboard Training Conference papers a few years back where a child is asked, after the assistant puts a vertical line on the chalkboard of 4 or 5 inches, to proceed to place the alphabet on the chalkboard, alternating sides, anyway he wishes but alternating sides. We'll find children reversing letters, omitting letters of the alphabet, sometimes 2 and 3 of them, misplacing letters of the alphabet, all kinds of things. Where with the same child, when you ask him to say the alphabet or write the alphabet or in any other wise produce the alphabet, now has no problem handling it. There's something of a differential here—simply this business of moving from one side to another. Of being able to deal with a spatial relationship, of a movement nature that isn't even labeled right and left, and yet is a right and left move, that he has problems dealing with on the motor level and comes out with these visual perceptual difficulties in the alphabet. Reversing of the "Z" is very common. Reversing of the "J" is also common. To see the "U" come after the "Q" is not uncommon, or to see the "U"-"V" left out is not uncommon, or other inconsistencies. Or to see a child that's absolutely unable to deal with this thing and just peter right out after he gets about half of it done. He's just bushed, absolutely bushed in doing it. This one we've only been doing for the past year to two years. We don't try to make an awful lot out of it other than what I've told you, just to see what happens.

Lecture III

We have been talking about trying to communicate some of the information that we can gather in the visual examination to the parent who isn't familiar with our particular way of observing and who isn't familiar with our particular vocabulary. One of the things that has begun to happen, infrequently but it has begun to happen, is a reverse of this where the parents begin to come in, communicating to us, having been communicated to by an educator in our terms; in terms of our observations and in terms of our language that they understand, behavioral language. I point this out because of the educator's guide and checklist. We have had children come in with the check list filled out by the teacher about the child without our having given it to the parent. Teachers, educators and people in education are beginning to pick this kind of material up and are utilizing it to direct the parents to the proper source of visual appraisal. If you are not using the educator's guide and check list, use it. Send two of them home with the next child in, one for the parent to keep, to evaluate, to assess the child against, and the other one to be sent to the classroom teacher of the child for return to you as she fills out the checklist.[2]

I will now talk about the last item on our pre-training testing that I didn't quite get to. What we do with this, from a 1st grader right on through, whether it's school age or adult, is to hand a 3 x 5 card with

---
2. *Editor's note: The Educator's Guide to Classroom Vision Problems with the checklist continues to be an excellent resource to use to get input from educators and is available from OEP directly or through the on-line store at www.oepf.org.*

Fewer Fatal Failures are the Result of Years of Scientific Study Combined with the Experience of Years.

this material typed on it to the patient and say, "Would you please count the 'f's'."

That's what I'm going to ask you the reader to do. Take some time and count the f's and then we'll have some fun with it maybe. We do this even with the 1st grader or the non-reading child because if you will recall, my instructions to you were not to read this but to count the "f's". Let me ask you some questions. How many of you counted 3 fs in this, only 3. Would you raise your hands? (1 person) How many counted 4, raise your hands? All right, we have a sizable group. How many counted 5 "f's"? More. How many counted 6 "f's"? More How many counted 7 "f's"? How many counted 8 "f's"? (1 person) Good. I have never had a group yet that counted 8 "f's". But I have yet to see a group, from a group as small as perhaps 18 to 20, to 150 to 200 count all the same on this apparently simple task that you would expect a 1st grader to do, because they do teach 1st grade children how to identify an "f". We have some problem here I think, if we are counting anywhere from 3 to 4 to 5 to 6 to 7 "f's" in a sophisticated group like yourselves. But seriously, what do you think we're looking at here? How could we have such a disparity in the counting of those "f's"?

There are some of you who did not see to count any of the "f's" in the 3 small words "of". How many of you didn't see any of those "f's" at all? Let's see it, because there are going to be many of you. In fact, there are going to be at least 2 to 3 times as many of you who missed these than who actually counted them. Maybe a few of you missed the "f'" that was imbedded in the word "scientific"? You all got the 3 big "F's" at the top, I'm sure. But what happens is, something to do I think with the inter-sensory organization of visual-auditory-verbal integrations. That we can look at a letter and because we are sophisticated perhaps, do more hearing of what we're seeing than seeing of what we're seeing. What is happening is that we scan right over the thing and not even identify it for the strictly visual aspects of the thing, because it's so embedded in the auditory or the verbal aspects of it. The sound of that "f" in those words is a "v", not an "f" and it thus it wasn't seen as an "f".

I don't try necessarily to make any particular diagnosis on the fact that the child or the adult doesn't read all of the "f's". However, what we have tended to see is with the very young child who is practically non-reading—and this could be even 3rd grade or so—who tends to count all of the "f's", who comes up with 7 on this, Generally speaking, I think we have a more difficult problem with this case. He tends to have a poorer relationship going for him already on symbol sound association. It's too easy for him to see the visual aspect of the thing but too hard for him to make the match between that and the auditory. This seems to be what we observe. When we get into the older youngsters and the adults, I think we have a different situation. We have possibilities there, as I see it at this point anyway. That is, some of us have such highly developed skills for visual identification that we can switch our gears and we can proofread, looking for the "f", or we can scan and pick up the information without necessarily seeing all of it. And since I did ask you to count the "f's", I didn't ask you to read it, some of you did just that. Some of you did just count the "f's" and came up with the 7. On the other hand, some of you, even though I said just count the "f's", I'm sure you spent more energy reading it than looking for the "f's" and therefore missed out on some of the "f's." In other words, it's a pretty slippery kind of situation if you're thinking in terms of diagnosing on the basis of it. But it does give you some idea of how the individual is utilizing his visual auditory system in a verbal matching kind of way. Does he listen to the instructions? Does he do what you've asked? Is he capable of doing it? And just what kind of a number he comes up with.

We've seen in some instances—in one case very recently of a youngster who counted 7 "f's", about 3 months ago at the end of the 10th session when we reintroduced this particular test, he counted 5 "f's." We had made significant gains with this child. This is the same child I have already mentioned. But here is the child who had been on megavitamin therapy for 2 months prior to our training by Dr. Allan Cott in New York City and responded very favorably, very quickly, much more so in time than I would have anticipated for the amount of visual problem we have found. I at least feel I can attribute this to the kind of medical treatment he was having prior to the training and during the training. This is the boy who at the end of the 10 weeks no longer counted 7 "f's," and this is the boy who the teacher also said, as reported by the parents on that last visit, "It's like a different child in the classroom." I feel sometimes that not counting them can be better than counting.

All right, let's go on, because what we're going to do now is just as the program says, "Developing the Home Assistant." However, this hour and the next hour of "Making Home Assignments Relevant" are really a blend. You don't make full use of the home assistant with-out making the home assignments relevant. We'll be talking about these two things kind of together. I'm going to do this, or try to do it at least, around a series of activities that we utilize in the office and at home, that we expose the parents to, that we may expose the child to, and that I may expose myself to in front of the parent. But we do not hesitate to ask the parent to participate in these activities. In fact, this is one of the critical things; to let the parent recognize that things, which on the surface may appear to be relatively simple or easy, may not at all be that simple, especially as the instructions become more complex or there are more activities or pieces of information to deal with.

Let's talk about the first one. The first one on the activity sheets as you see them here are in the format that we use for home assignments. When an activity is assigned at home, it's discussed with the parent. It's discussed verbally and the parent has this sheet in front of him. The parent then takes this activity sheet home with any specific notes that might have been made on it, any additional information or alteration to fit more particularly the particular child we're dealing with, so that it is more or less tailored for their own needs at home. This particular one is also done the day it's assigned for home. It's done in the office in the presence of the parents with the child. It's done with the child by one of my assistants, as I am working with the parents. It's kind of a family situation and it's not uncommon for both of the parents to be present during the training session in the area that the training is done in conversation with me while they're getting instruction. They aren't told this in advance that they're going to be getting a 5-hour workshop seminar-oriented kind of training, but they are told that I'll be spending time with them. But this is literally what they get—a workshop session with their own child, where they also participate in some of the things they'll be working with their child at home.

This first one is; "Ball on String with Body Participation - To and Fro - phase 1." There's another one that I'll just mention on the next page where it's the same idea but Rotating; phase 2. But this particular one in phase 1, we do this to help the parent recognize how predictive the visual system is in what the child is going to do with this ball activity. We use a Marsden ball setup. The assistant takes the ball, moves it back, asks the child to stand with his hands spread apart, about one foot to two feet apart, so that the ball when it's released, will wind up at about his chest level. He's asked to catch the ball from the side. We point out to the parent, the reason we're asking him to do this is that we want him to be very aware of the predictive role of vision in this catching of the ball. We used to see too many children stand there, catching the ball, before we asked them to move their hands apart, with a flinch, with a turning-aside of their head, with a closing of the eyes, or with the various other things that you'll see, or with this jarring shudder of surprise when the ball finally lands in their hands, and it's a jolt all over but they've got it. This is a kind of tactual surprise to the visual system. He's able to deal with it but he isn't predicting very well when the event will happen.

So what we want him to do is to recognize this first, so he holds his hands out and the ball is released. If he doesn't make a decent visual prediction of the ball and where it is, then it hits him before he gets his hands to it, or his hands are out there too soon and it bounces off, or you can see him recognizing that his predictions aren't going right and he gets his hands out there well ahead of the ball to stop it. So we talk to him about it again, we want him to catch it from the sides. We may talk to him about using his fingertips even, just to get his hands on the sides of the ball. Once he does this, then we ask him, "This time, you can start pushing the ball when we let it go. Push it back." The assistant usually stands out there and says, "Push it towards me." What we want him to do now is to maintain still this high order of visual predictiveness of where the ball is, so we say, "Touch it gently." At the same time, he will be aware of where the assistant is out there to push it in a straight line. So, you're dealing with these two aspects of visual space simultaneously—the touching of the ball gently here and the awareness of where it's going to go out there with the thrust. If he does one of these rather well but loses the awareness of the space relationships, as they frequently will do, he may hit the ball gently but the ball will go off course. When we draw his attention to the direction that the ball is now going in, he may be able to get it back on course but he begins hitting the ball hard in the near area. This indicates to me that he's shifting awareness from one area to another area. What we're looking for is the simultaneous awareness of the visually predictive movements internally for handling both of these areas of space simultaneously.

I will frequently point out to the parents, since this is perhaps the 3rd week that we will introduce this particular one- -that this is not too dissimilar from the child's demand tasks in the classroom of copying work from chalkboard to desk where he has to maintain relationships of what he's doing out there with what he's doing down here. This may very well have been the child who demonstrates that he's handling either the contact on the ball gently or the direction but not the two things at the same time, with a history of having had difficulty in copying work accurately. But here we put him now into a concrete situation where he has immediate feedback and immediate consequence and we can help him to develop some immediate awareness of the results of his own lack of consistency in prediction. So that normally, even within the demonstration in the office this first time out with it, we can see a change in a matter of a couple of minutes from not even being able to get his hands on it to now, a couple of minutes later, pushing it in a straight line and touching it gently. There seem to be an awful lot of the marbles that are there and it doesn't often seem to be too difficult to begin to help him put them together if we can break the pieces down to see where the original difficulty seems to be.

We're not satisfied with this. As you read the activity sheet, you'll see some of the several other things that we ask him to do. These things are usually very enlightening, both to the parent and to us, because any good training program, as you well know, is a continuing testing program. We couldn't possibly, as I've described in my approach to the testing situation, have explored all of the areas that I would be interested in going into the training program. The training program continues to be an observational testing program as we go. The next question we ask this child is, now that he has been able maybe to alternate hands and use both hands together or just use the right and just use the left and keep it going straight and contact gently, is, "Would you now tap the floor with your foot as you touch the ball with your hand." This is where we see some more breakdowns in performance. What will frequently happen is a tremendous amount of intensity in his own movement patterns—the foot will hit the floor and you'd swear he's going to go through the floor if he could; it's so hard, so intense. The same thing happens to the ball. The course goes off. It's as though his awareness of what he is doing now has been so centered on what his hand and foot are doing, that it's as though he's reading or monitoring much less of the space world around him. But this isn't what we want. We want him to be able to monitor his own internal space world and this external space world simultaneously. This is the way we process information most effectively. This is the way we set our own gears for action, for information processing more effectively. What we would do, we would simply stop the ball and we would ask him, "Did you still touch it gently? Did it go in a straight line?" We make no judgments on it, we ask him to. If there's going to be a judgment, we ask him to make it for himself immediately. Not after he's done it several times, but immediately the assistant stops the ball and asks the question.

The other kind of response we see here immediately is, aside from a good response, the child who still monitors what's going on out here with his hand pretty well. He's still touching it fairly gently and he's still pushing it in a pretty good straight line, but what we hear is a mismatch in timing between the contact of the ball and hand and the contact of the floor and foot. It would be hand usually first—not always but more often than not. Immediately again the assistant stops the ball and asks the child the question, "What did you touch first, the ball or the floor? Can you tell?" Usually there's a dead silence. She may ask another question, 'Did you feel your hand on the ball or your foot on the floor first? Did you hear the sound of the hand on the ball or the sound of the foot on the floor first?" She's trying to awaken in him these ever-present systems that are potentially able to monitor his own actions and his own operations. He's thinking so highly of what his hand is doing and what his foot is doing and what he's seeing there that he no longer hears a relationship between what happened. He no longer feels the relationship between what happened. But if we can stop the activity immediately and ask him these questions, we'll find sometimes it seems like an eternity—it may be only 10 or 15 or 20 seconds but it will seem like an eternity. You can see the parents getting a little itchy. You know, "What are you trying to do to him like this?" And he'll come up with the right answer. It's as though it takes him forever to reprocess, to put it through again, to put all the pieces together, to assemble it, and by golly, he can come up and tell you what has happened. "Yes, I felt my hand on the ball," or, "My hand hit the ball first and then my foot." It doesn't always happen on the first try. Sometimes the first try, when we ask this kind of question of him—to sit back and take a look at the actions or the result of the processes that he used, it is merely apparently to help him to awaken the possibilities of still listening while he's doing it, or still feeling while he's doing it. It may take a couple or three times before he begins to even be able to respond to you.

But I can't help but think of these kids in the classroom with the relentlessness of reading and of the goal approach attitude in the average classroom, that this child seldom has an opportunity exposed to him to sit back and take a look at what he's just done, to find out then and there and now what he has just done. And then and there and now, to take another opportunity to see if he can reestablish or rearrange or reorder or in another point of view handle this particular set of activities. You will frequently find this child, when he does begin to reorder his eye-hand-foot organization, his internal space and listening so he's monitoring and he can come up and tell us that he's monitoring, that he still now begins to lose the external world again. He loses control of the ball. So again we stop it and ask him—we go back and forth between his awareness of the internal, his awareness of the external. So that in time, and usually it doesn't take an awful lot of time doing it this way, he begins to be able to deal with what's going on internally with this prediction of what he wanted to do out there.

There are some other variations that we will use with this. We have used this kind of thing in workshop demonstrations, using optometrists as subjects and we find we get many different kinds of responses within our own group. It's not just with the child. But this is one of the ones that we would demonstrate with the child so that the parent can begin to get some insight of this point of view of asking the child some questions about what they observed in his behavior. It's a very interesting phenomenon, the changing attitude that you can begin to recognize with some of the parents of these children where the parents have been rather hardnosed about what they expected of their child, when they can see this kind of processing going on and see a result from it. They begin to back off a little bit, too. They begin to take a different approach to their own child in a learning situation and help him move along a heck of a lot faster.

Let's go on to the activity sheet— "Cross Pattern Walking with Flashlights." With this, what we're doing is simply adding a visual orientation to the cross pattern walking. We use flashlights a great deal with most of these youngsters to give them an immediate consequence, once again, of their own operations and of their own actions. This particular activity, which we will frequently assign the first week—I would say that as many as 90% of the cases that we will work within these areas that we're talking about, will have this as the first-week assignment. It's the first opportunity that we've perhaps had to put one of the activities into the hands of the parents so that the parents begin to feel this. I usually demonstrate. What I do, I take the flashlights—and I'll get at one end of the examination area and start walking cross pattern, shining the right light on the left foot, the left light on the right foot and just walk smoothly, easily, shining the light on the shoe. The light is on the shoe—that's part of the instructions. I do this; I walk back and forth, and then hand the lights to the parents and ask them to do the same thing. I would say that in 75% of the cases, the parents/will not be able to start out very well. They'll take a misstep with the right foot and right hand and sometimes continue that way, not realizing that this isn't what I said. Or they will take a step or two and realize it and then stop and kind of laugh. Or they will walk right on down, and shining the light over to the left side, miss the foot by anywhere from 6 inches to 3 feet for the whole length of the room. When they get to the end of the room, I'll say, "How many times did the light shine on your foot?" Most of them-here we get another smile because they are able to monitor it if you give them time to, rather than say, "You didn't do it right," we say, "Did you see it?" And most of them recognize that they didn't see the light on the foot. So we say, "Try it again?" I do it purposely, I say "Try it again and this time make sure the light goes on the foot." I put them a little tighter on center visually. What happens invariably with the parent when he does this is that his walking stiffens and he's getting the light on the foot. We ask them, "Did you notice something happened to the way you were walking, to your whole body?" I ask them, "What was the difference in what you were doing?" You were looking harder, you were monitoring and making a better match there but it jammed up other things. If you're going to try to learn under these conditions, you're not going to learn very efficiently or very well. When your body is as tight and stressed as it was while you were doing that, do you think you'd like to sit down and read? Do you think you'd like to sit down and solve a problem or communicate with your husband, or your wife, if you're feeling like this? You wouldn't, you'd rather go on out and walk it off."

If we have to teach a child to learn under these conditions, I think we're kind of going down the wrong alley. What we point out is, "All right, now that you're aware of it, you can begin to do something about it. Now let's try it again, but this time begin to be aware of your internal world, loosen up and try to walk the way you walked before but keep looking." They can do it just like their children can do it. But the point is, they have to go through this kind of thing themselves before they can fully understand what the child is going to have to go through. Sometimes a sharp optometrist will come to me afterwards about this and ask, "What kind of parents are these? College graduates? How did they become college graduates? How did they achieve? How did they perform if they couldn't do this?" And some of the parents pick this kind of thing up. I remember one parent—in Latham, N.Y., we're about 4 miles north of Albany, this is within a couple of hours of the Adirondacks or the Catskill Mountains or the Berkshires or the Green Mountains of Vermont and there's a lot of skiing in the area, as there probably is out here. We have people who live north of us who will come in sometimes having picked everybody off the ski slopes to make it down to the office in time, still in their ski togs. I remember one woman who had one devil of a time with this cross pattern walking, trying to get it organized and trying to free up. Her body stiffened in such a way that she would never have been able to ski like that. She said afterwards—because she picked this thing up herself—"How come I can ski so well?" I said, "I don't know. I have no idea, except I would have one other question. How much better might you be able to ski if you had these kinds of organizations under control?" And that's the only question I can say about it. This is what we're trying to do, help them begin to monitor more of their potential so that they can work from still a broader base.

This is why I love to work with children who are already achieving. Because I think we can help them achieve still further and closer to their potential. Just because we're doing well doesn't necessarily mean we're approaching potential. This is the point of view that we take. We want them to explore their potentials and their abilities to deal with things. When we're working with a group in a workshop or in a demonstration with a group like this when we get volunteers, I would now have asked for a second group of volunteers and I would have said to them, "You saw what the others did. We're going to start from there and now I'm going to ask you to name your hand or foot as you walk. I say that means you're to start naming the hand that's shining the light. It would be left, right. It would be the hand shining the light out front. Or if I said 'foot', it would be the foot that has the light on it out in front. But I only want you to name it four times—right, left, right, left—then stop, but keep walking. They haven't gone through the feelings of just the sheer movements of looking at their own walking pattern that they've used for 20, 30, 40, 50, or 60 years. They've used it every day, but they haven't stopped to look at it to see how it's organized. Now they start out walking and I say, "Hands." Some of them stop dead in their tracks, others will keep going and get all mixed up with the lights. The lights will start swinging off their feet and their bodies will be stiffening up. Others will not be able to do the naming but they'll keep walking. There are so many possibilities. I've seen in one instance an optometrist walking with the right foot forward and his right arm thrust toward the left, shining those lights like so (illustrating), and there was something about it—clinically, you can just tell that when you talk to this man while he's still moving and doing this and get him to become aware of what he's doing, He's just as apt to fall over on his ear. So I did it anyway while he was walking and I stayed a little bit behind with my arm around, not touching him, and asked him if the light was shining on the foot. Is his right hand swinging for-ward with his left foot? When he became aware of it, he did, he toppled.

We cannot always monitor all of these systems simultaneously. It would be nice if we could and could do this all the time but we must be careful on how we do it, so we work gradually on things like this. This is why I use the second group and I would normally only do it with optometrists where I would load them. Sometimes, depending upon the nature of the parents we're working with, we unload them because some of them have to be loaded like this before they really get the feel of what their job is as assistants for that child at home, because that's whom they're assistants for, for their child. They have to understand something about him in order to help him, in order to be an assistant for him. With this kind of parent who needs a little more convincing, we'll put the lights in their hands and ask them right at the outset to do all these things.

The other thing that happens, incidentally, that I didn't mention is that if they do get this thing going maybe right, left, right, left, they just keep right on going, "right, left," several times until they stop walking or until I tell them to stop walking and then they stop talking. I'll say, "How many times did you say 'right, left'?" Remember I had asked them to do it four times? "Oh, I forgot all about it." "This is the same kind of thing that happens to your child. He forgets sometimes, too, when we give him too many bits of information all at once, when we give him too many things to handle all at once and he's not quite ready to handle some of these pieces." We will find out how much he can handle, and this is all we want to give him right now. Once he can organize this and begin to deal with this, then we'll give him one more bit of information that requires some other monitoring or some other awareness or some other aspect of the activity. But we will build it in this way so that he can continue to perform and achieve at the activity. We don't want to give him too many things to do all at once.

These activities—the next one being "Child in Mirror"—are not arranged in any particular sequence as we would use them in the office or one following another at all. These are simply some activities that I've pretty much selected at random that do help to communicate some of the notions and some of the concepts that we would like the parents to take home with them, to begin to work with the child. For example, on this particular one Child in Mirror, we would normally be doing this with most of these children maybe not until the 5th or 6th week, it just depends. Some of them we would be doing it earlier if the child has already demonstrated an ability to deal with his own rights and lefts in our testing, and he can still deal with his rights and lefts while he's in movement—because that's a different activity again—the child who runs into trouble naming his hands and feet while he's walking, may not have trouble naming his hands and feet if he's standing still. It's simply how much can he monitor. How much can he move into cortical activity and thinking processes and see that things are going right and balance and posture and all of these things all at once. If he's been demonstrating that he can handle this kind of thing, then we would go to "Child in Mirror".

The basic idea here is to give him an activity dealing with rights and lefts that he must manipulate. He must do some thinking about it while he's looking. I do want him in a visual environment to do this thing. What we're going to ask him to do is to play with the labels. He's going to look in the mirror, a full-length mirror if possible at home, and look at this little boy in front of him and make believe that this little boy in the mirror is a robot. He's going to be able to tell this little boy what to do, how to move. That the little boy in the mirror can't do things for himself, he has to be told. The idea then would be for him to say to the boy in the mirror, as an example, "Wave to me with your right hand." This assumes that he's able to see the transformation and in his own organization raise his left hand and wave to the boy in the mirror while he's seeing the boy in the mirror wave with his right hand. It's very often that a parent will pick up a possibility here and say, "Won't this confuse him?" I'm very quick to say, "Yes, it may confuse him if he isn't ready for it." The readiness deals with this transformation, this spatial transformation. I point out to the parent how to help him take that step, because by this time I have had some evidence that I think he's ready for it, and it's rarely we find that they come back at the end of the week that he hasn't been able to solve this operation by the end of the week.

But we help the parent with the child who is having more difficulty with it, or is more apt to by saying, "Stand alongside of him as he stands before the mirror and raise your hand like this and ask him which hand is this that you've just raised. If he can name that as your right hand, say, "Fine, that's my right hand." Watch where it goes, watch what happens to it, as I tell the parent to turn around alongside the mirror now and ask the child, "Which hand is that?" If he says, "Right," he's got the transformation. If he says, "Left," he's still not seeing this transformation and we may do it again. We say, "Put something in your hand, an apple, a ball, a piece of chalk. Which hand is holding the chalk? Does my other hand have any chalk in it?" "No." "Which hand is holding the chalk?" And do it gradually, and see if he can begin to recognize that there is a shifting or this transformation in our world and that our labels have to match these transformations; that our labels are very flexible things anyway. They're culturally induced. In France it would be *droit*, not right. It's just a sound label for this particular side, not even this particular hand or this particular movement or this particular direction or from another point of view in that direction, depending upon one's point of view. That it's a very flexible thing and must be able to be manipulated if it's going to be dealt with efficiently. The child is asked to do this in the classroom, not necessarily to get up and recite about it, but in his reading he goes in this direction but the teacher faces him in that direction, so there's her right and her left while this is his left and his right. He has these inconsistencies, if this is what they are. But we want him now to manipulate this at a thinking level while he's looking at these actions and movements. They can usually begin to do this.

Then of course, you can make it a little bit more complicated by moving two parts, touching the right knee with the left hand. We also have found that if the parent tells the child what to do, generally speaking, this is more difficult. Generally speaking, the child finds it easier if he can originate these directions, these instructions to the robot from an internal feeling of what he's going to do rather than the parent seeing, "Have the boy in the mirror raise his right hand."

If you think of the differential in process here, that's auditory, it must be projected back out there, a transformation to the right side of the robot back to his own side, now I'll raise my left hand. Where the other way, I may have the feeling here I want to have him move that, feeling this match, and now that's my left, have him move his right. It's a different process entirely. So we have them do it both ways. On very few occasions, we'll find a child who will do it easier from the auditory input than from his own feelings. We think in terms of flexibility. We'd like him to be able to handle these things in many ways.

One other point about this type of an activity and about, generally speaking, the programming itself, I did state yesterday that we assign activities each week. Each week they get a new set of activities. Normally, we assign about five activities for each weekly workout. Each week there may very well be some activity that will make some kind of demand on this laterality, directionality organization. But it will be on a different kind of activity. We hope that the child is going to be able to draw some relationships between these activities from week to week. This is part of the relevancy too, in the training program, to be able to deal with the same concept from another point of view; to be able to deal with the same activity with some other possibilities of seeing something else in it. We do the same with all these activities.

For my own purposes, I break the activities down into a category of gross motor, identification, pursuit, saccadic, eye-hand, and visualization. Under any of these categories—in fact, this particular one is under visualization—the cross pattern walking with flashlights is under gross motor. But under any of these circumstances, you see, he may use a gross motor activity that has a very high intensity, a component that is visualization, or that requires a considerable amount of movement pattern at a thinking level, no less at the motor level. So we do try to broaden each of the activities; whether I've labeled it pursuit or saccadic for identification into other movement patterns and into other types of awareness. Therefore, at the end of the 10 weeks that we'd normally build this kind of thing, the parents have developed a considerable idea of our approach. By the end of this time, they can go back to the 1st activities and use them again, but now differently because they have changed as well as the child.

They can begin to ask other questions that would require a little bit more sophistication on the part of the child, a little bit more elaboration, to be able to listen, to be able to communicate while he's doing the activity. To listen to other instructions, a question that may have no relationship at all to the activity he's engaged in and then this kind of questioning, "Can he communicate about something completely unrelated to the activity he's engaged in?" Or does the activity stop? A lot of the children, even well along in the training program, you'll find this is a necessity for them. If they're going to listen, they have to stop all other action, all other systems. It's the child behind the phoropter who, when you ask him questions, he pulls his head away, "What do you mean?" Or he pulls his head away and says, "What did you say?" while he's looking at you. Unless he has you in visual view, he finds it difficult—and unless he centers on you visually, he finds it difficult to deal with auditory processing.

It's by pointing these possibilities out to the child and to the parents that they then have many opportunities to deal with it. You take a situation like this dealing with the rights and lefts of the mirror activity. The father of the boy I've described who was on megavitamin therapy who responded so favorably with the visual training and that megavitamin therapy, I think came in for about 2 of these 10 sessions, only. The man was very sharp in terms of picking up the ideas, and his wife must have been communicating to him pretty well, but it happened to be the day that we assigned either this activity or another one that had this kind of manipulative aspect to laterality directionality. The following week, the mother in describing the reaction to the activity at home and the child's response to it, said, "And do you know what my husband did? He sent the boy into the dining room to set the table and as he set the table on one side, my husband said, 'Don't go around to the other side, but set it now from the side you're on.'" With a family like this who begin to pick up these concepts, begin to pick up these notions, they begin to expand the whole thing into so many other things. This is what I think of in terms of arranging conditions for learning. That we have spread the notions, the ideas that we have to someone else's thinking who can now begin to direct and arrange some conditions in another environment outside of our office.

This is the kind of thing also that those school systems which have incorporated optometric thinking have been able to do as well.

Lecture IV

Let's move on to "Coding at the Chalkboard". This particular activity is one of those things that happened to us, the testing that I mentioned yesterday that we have extracted from Abe Kirschner on visual count, auditory count, tactile count, and kinesthetic count. We ran into some questions on this when we started doing the testing. We found children who weren't able to monitor these things, weren't able to handle these things. What do we do about it? There are a number of things that would come to mind but this is one of the things that came to mind, and we've seen some very interesting things; not just with the Brock String type of thing with two strings, I just want something else. What I ask him to do as he does this is to look at the tack but to be aware of the string. That's a very simple thing. Some of those parents stop moving the pencil, some of them stop looking at the tack and start looking at the string. But this is the point, and we want them to go through this to hear these mismatches in the instructions as they've been given to what they are doing, so that they realize it. This helps them then to look at this same sort of performance with the child, so that the child can begin to look at something. But be aware of something else, to be aware of the relationship that exists between the thing he's looking at and other space in the volume around it. The first thing is, look at the tack and be aware of the string. When they can do that and still keep it moving, not start going like this (illustrating)—all kinds of things happen with movement even. If it doesn't stop, it may go too fast, so you get them to be aware that their movement has changed. You just do it slowly, keep looking at the tack and have them be aware of the string.

Then I ask them, "Do you notice a changing relationship between the tack and the string?" Sometimes you may see the string to the right or left of the tack, sometimes above or below the tack." We get some parents who will say, "No, Dr., it's always below the tack." Here we have a point of communication on the basis of a point of view that I think what this parent is telling me is that what they are communicating to me about the string is not the string itself but the point of attachment of the string, and that's different. I didn't say the point of attachment of the string was changing to the right or to the left, or that the point of attachment of the string was above or below. I'll agree with the parent. I'll say, "Yes, I think you may be right. The string at that end is always below the tack." I'll say, "What were you thinking about in terms of the string?" And many of them will be able to say, "Yes, I was talking about." And then they'll say, "Oh." As one woman said the other day, "There's another end." And I said, "Yes, and there's something in between. That's the string." And really, this is the way vision goes sometimes perceptually, that we see pieces and we don't always get all the pieces back together again, even though we can see the whole situation, they don't go together in the same order.

There are all kinds of demonstrations with your tachistoscope, with the Lyons and Lyons series, on the "P" series particularly where you have them reproduce some of these things, maybe two arrows, and they have made the rotation in space very accurately. Except they did it on an individual basis rather than the whole picture basis, and when they put them together, they didn't go together right. Maybe I said that too fast. This one particularly, we've seen it. (illustrating) Ask them to rotate it 90 degrees clockwise, for example, and they rotate it like this. You can spend half a training session sometimes just getting something out of a thing like this of how it happened, what they did. Can they begin to cross monitor their own process? Begin to see what they did themselves? They took a piece of the form and rotated just that piece, instead of rotating the whole thing at one time. That they did it in pieces and put the pieces back together again and the pieces didn't go together the same way they started out, they didn't see or understand that our perceptual field, visual organization can be like this. What we're trying to do here with the parent and child this week is to help him see these relationships as a solid ground base in a total volume and space. Because this is where the questions first begin—look at the tack and be aware of the string. Can they now see the string projected off to the left, or off to the right, or above or below? This is not an easy task for some of these people. It's awfully hard for them to *see* that string anywhere but below the tack, until they can begin to open up. This is a volume you're talking about, not a plane out here where the string is attached to the pencil with the tack; you're talking about the whole space here.

We would then ask them another question that sometimes really shakes them up. We'll say, "Take a look at the string now. You see it? You see how long it is? Put it up again and do this again. Does the string always look the same length?" No, it doesn't. "Does it always feel the same length?" This is where you get, "'No, it doesn't even feel the same length sometimes—it feels longer, sometimes it feels shorter." I said, "Did you notice any of those things before I asked the question?" "No, I didn't notice any of those things." There are so many things that may be mismatched within our own organization of the meaningfulness of the things we're dealing with out here that we move on as though it were as it is; without its being as it is, without any awareness that we are seeing it so differently from the fellow next to us. But we don't always see it the same way or understand it the same way or see the same relationships in the same way, or deal with as much volume in the same way as the fellow next to us. What we're interested in right now in communicating with the parent so that they can become a good assistant at home, is to let them recognize that when the teacher sits there with 30 kids in that classroom and she says something or does something or expresses something or demonstrates something, that their little guy may be one of the kids that saw this thing or heard this thing in some way that's no relationship to the way the teacher intended it. We would like to have them and their child in a better position to accept a point of view and to recognize possibilities in situations; especially in this visual area.

The next question we ask the parents is—we will point out to them, "In doing this now, you are aware of something that you weren't aware of before. The chances are, as you reprocess this and do this, that you'll begin to find that there will be a difference, that you won't always feel it different. You will see it differently because the visual inputs don't always give you all of the information that you need. What we are working with here is the visual information, what you already know about it because you have picked it up and felt it and looked at it so you went; right to it and thought you saw it all. We would simply like you to be able to recognize that you don't see it all even though you know it all. We want you to put the pieces together and to recognize where the information comes from; some of it is from prior experience of having seen it in another position in space, and recognize you're not always seeing it in the same position in space." I don't know how much value some of these points are, but it's been a positive enough situation in getting information across to a lay person who has no basis or background or knowledge in perception or vision or spatial organization or the kinds of experiences that are necessary in order to abstract meaning from symbols that it gives us some kind of a communication where we begin to understand one another. From this, I think we really do begin to understand one another.

The third question we would ask after this seeing of change of relationship, feeling of the possibilities of differences in feeling and seeing, and yet knowing at the same time that it isn't different, we would then say, "Can you see the rest of the room?" Let me tell you of an experience we had in our study group one night when we did this with one of the men. He dropped the pencil, the string and the tack to the floor and grabbed the arms of the chair. He was seated, he wasn't even standing. He was fine up to that point, he was beginning to see these relationships and he was dealing with this information up in here. And when I asked him about the rest of the room, he dropped it and he turned color, I'm not exaggerating, he turned color. I don't know what color it was; it was some kind of a grayish-greenish something-or-other. When he could talk about it afterwards, the only explanation he had for it was that he wasn't sure whether he was falling off the chair or the room was going around, and he wasn't real sure. He grabbed onto the chair. I have not ever had that radical of an experience with any parent to this day.

Most of the really severe reactions we've had have been with optometrists. They really make good subjects. What I'd like you to do here is to see something that we do with the parent when the parent can report to us that they have seen something in the room moving, shifting—maybe the light fixture on the ceiling, or maybe me, or maybe a desk across the room, or an instrument stand moving. I say, "Would you now point to it." Let's do this, everybody, just with your thumb. Hold your thumb up—you can do it binocularly, we won't even bring you down to the monocular level. But hold it out free and easy, don't tighten it up. Just look at your thumb, go around in a circle. Got your eye on your thumb, really looking at it? Are you aware of the rest of the room? Is the room stable? How many say the room is stable? How many say there's a lot of motion in the room? I'm going to talk to all you people who see motion in the room. Let's try something. Those of you who saw something move, can you select some item from this environment that was in motion while you were looking at your thumb and point to it with your other hand. Now, put your other thumb up that you were following before. Look at your thumb and move it in a circle but keep pointing at the thing that was moving. How many of you now find that the thing that was moving is no longer moving? Good. How many of you find that the thing that was moving is still moving? There are going to be some. I think this is a little more embeddedness, as I think of it, at least.

The question that you should ask of yourselves is, "Why should the thing that was moving this way, no longer move this way?" Does it happen to a lot of you? "What effect did putting my hand out here and pointing in a direction in space have upon the things that I saw?" Our parents see it happen to them, the kids see it happen to them, and I've never talked to an optometric group that couldn't see it happen. And I've never talked to an optometric group where we asked about it that we didn't find some who continued to see it happen. If you want to explore it, what you do? You start chasing the things that are moving. And incidentally, in training, this is why we want to do this with the two circuits, because I'm not the least bit convinced that the two circuits are going to handle these things in the same way unless they have an opportunity to at least make an attempt to see what it's like with the right eye, the left eye, and then with the two eyes together. But try it. If something moves over there, point to it. Now something moves over there, point to it, something moves up here, point to it. Some of you are going to see, as soon as you begin to do this, the whole thing is going to be stable out there, just with a few pointings. There will no longer be motion. This would not be true with my friend in the study group who thought he was falling off the chair. It would take a lot longer with him.

Let's move on. The next activity sheet in here is "Space Matching.[3]" Space matching is an activity that I use, certainly for training at

---

3. *This procedure is similar to "Estimating Distances" as taught as part of the OEP Clinical Curriculum*

home, but there is communication value in it for the parent. This is essentially what I'm talking to you about. These are just any old activity, but how we communicate some of the way of dealing with a situation to parents who may not have been accustomed to handling their child in this way. What this activity asks is, "Tell me, Johnny, how many steps it will take for you to go from where you are to that table." In the office, I generally use a door as a reference because I'm going to make an illustration. I'll say, if he was standing here and I asked him, "How many steps to go to the door?" Think, Mother, how different this would be if I said, "Johnny, go over and close the door," to "Johnny, how many steps will it take for you to go to the door, to close it, if you want?" But I'm asking him to become aware simultaneously of his internal organization and that space world out there; to make some kind of a judgment, some kind of an estimation of what kind of movement patterns are involved in this visual space. These are movement patterns that he has used for his 6, 8, 10 years or whatever, but to make some kind of a value judgment as to how many steps it's going to take. And now take them.

So he starts taking them. He says, "Ten steps." And he gets out there about six and you see him start to shrink these steps down to make it, or stretch them out to make it fit. And boy, at that time I tell that mother, "If he does that and you see him do that, you say, "Hey, that's great! What did you do then? What did you see different then?"" This is what we're looking for, isn't it? We're looking for visual information to match up with our movement patterns, to match up with the other information so that it becomes more reliable and more consistent and more meaningful. And this is exactly what he's telling us, that somehow he saw it differently there than he did at the outset. Maybe he's saying, "I have to do a lot of moving before I can depend upon my movement patterns to match up with what I'm seeing." What I'd like him to be able to move to is the level where he no longer has to go through these movement patterns in order to know what he's seeing. He can match his movement patterns against his visual patterns without having to go through the actual operations.

This fits in the pattern of development, the kind of direction we'd like to see the visual process take so that it does become emergent and stand for these other operations so we no longer have to go through the kinds of movement patterns in order to get confirmation; that the visual system can stand for these things. If it can't stand for the physical factors and characteristics of the real concrete world around me, if I can't be consistent and understanding of these factors, what do I expect of the child when he's going to be trying to handle symbols; symbols of this physical world, symbols of abstractions of abstractions, when he can't handle at the physical level consistently? Let's give him an opportunity to begin to understand some of his own organization in his visual space relationships and then let him go off to these other things. He takes care of many of the other problems himself once he finds out what he's all about and how he relates to that world out there and how it relates to him. And incidentally, when he does see this and does begin to make these matches better, you'll find he's playing with the other kids better and that all of a sudden the other kids who haven't been playing with him and won't even let him play ball with them are picking him to be on their side. You know, kids can be real cruel. I suppose that's not a good word. Maybe I should say they are realists because they're not going to pick a child who they know isn't going to be able to make these spatial organizational relationships or matches with their own hands and feet. I'm sure they don't think about it that way. They say, "He's a clunk, that's all, he's a klutz. He can't catch the ball, he can't hit the ball." They're realists, and when the time comes a couple of months later that these same kids are picking this boy to play on the team, this is the kind of stuff the mothers tell me -- that the boy is now playing with the other kids, these kids are still the same realists. They recognize the difference in these children, in their playmates, in their peers, sometimes faster than we adults will. And we'll get into some of that on some of the philosophy of organizing these things in the next hour.

We don't always recognize some of the values ourselves nor do the people who are working with these children recognize the changes. It can really destroy your whole visual training program if you're not aware of it. What we get across to the parent here is, that for him to make a mid-course correction is no worse than the mid-course corrections they make when they go to the moon. If it's fair enough for the astronauts, it's fair enough for Johnny to make a change in his mind on his way, too. But we want him to be aware of it.

The next activity is, "Red and Green Balls on String." We came by these things as a fluke. We used to use a little jacks ball, one normally used for playing jacks. They had them at the Gesell Institute the year I was over there at their course and they had a source for these things and we used to buy them by the hundreds from the Institute and they bought them by the thousands. But they ran out of their source and couldn't get them anymore. We hunted and hunted and finally found a rubber company in Ohio, Barr Rubber,[4] that makes these little balls and we ordered a bunch of them, not knowing too much about it. But these red/green flame balls—as they are called—really are great with anaglyphs. They are just great with anaglyphs. This is what we use it for. When we get to the point where we have binocular matching and we have some consistency of information processing visually, we send them home now with this activity "Red and Green Balls on String." We also found a cordage company in Pawtucket, Rhode Island that made some nice shiny acrylic red and green string—twine. In fact, if you write to them at this point, you ask for optometric twine. They have it listed in their catalog this way, as optometric twine. It works beautifully also with the anaglyphs that we get from Bernell.[5] We send them home with this stuff and we put the green string on the red ball and the red string on the green ball and ask them to hold it. Now for the parents, what we do to get them initiated into this is simply, hold it in front of them while they look at it and then put the anaglyphs (red/green glasses) in front. Some of them will almost immediately begin to see something coming and going. Others are pretty good and they won't see anything suppressing until you start to move them. Others are even better, they won't see anything suppressing until they start to move them. Others are even better, they won't see anything suppressing until they stand up and look at it. Others are even better than that, they won't see anything suppressing until they bend over. Each one of these steps along the way, we have seen in optometric groups when we've been able to demonstrate it in workshop. They are going to go through the same kind of stages from sitting to eye movement, to standing, to standing with eye movement, to bending, to bending with eye movement. And all the way

---

4. *Editors Note: This company is no longer in business.*
5. *The original in the text was "Vodnoy," which refers to Dr. Bernard Vodnoy who began Bernell. Bernell Vision Therapy Product Company is located in Indiana.*

along, you'll find in that optometric group there will be an optometrist or two or a dozen who say, "Oh, oh, now it starts." All of these various changes in posture, gravitational, and reflex demands upon other systems can alter the effect on suppression. What I'm looking for, in pointing it out to the parents, we put them through it until we begin to see where the suppressions are, is that we would like to have a greater degree of consistency in this information processing; whether I happen to be in this position or in this position or in that position, or bending over to tie my shoe. This is something we would not send along until we had demonstrated it in the office and found he would be able to handle it.

"Parquetry - Phase 2" is the next activity. The concepts, the direction, the notion behind this, I heard described by Dr. Harry Wachs from Pittsburgh[6] at an Eastern Seaboard Training Conference[7] one year, several years back and it's probably in the transcript somewhere, I don't know just what year. The way we're using this now is, somewhere along in the training maybe by the 6th, 7th, or even the 8th week. We would ask the parent to observe this. We're going to use maybe the first two steps 1 and 2 the first time out. Steps 3 and 4 the 2nd time out, if steps 1 and 2 go all right. The next night we'll use Steps 5 and 6, and so on. We pair them off, in other words, and you'll see as you read it over later that one is the adverse of the other, in a sense.

Step 1, for example, would be for the parents to make a pattern of 3 or 4 parquetry blocks on a surface, a table surface, for the child to see. Then, under cover—like at a table here, we could put a chair under from the other side and that would be a table surface underneath the table. They now—the child reaches under, half of the parquetry set is there, and they reach down and feel without seeing the shapes of the blocks that are going to match the pattern that they have in front of them. So they put it together now, spatially, from what they see, without seeing what they are feeling. In other words, we're running information in the visual out through the tactual kinesthetic under the table.

---

6. *Dr. Wachs was from Pittsburgh at the time this presentation was given. At the time of publication Dr. Wachs lives in Maryland and has recently retired from practice in Washington DC.*
7. *This is the original name of the meeting called the Kraskin Invitational Skeffington Symposium on Vision, held every January in the Washington DC area.*

The second step would be just the reverse of this where the parent makes a pattern under cover, the child reaches under here and feels and then comes back up and puts together a visual match for what he felt. Some of you will see that there is other apparatus we use such as a cookie tin and play dough, this is for the children who have real trouble controlling their motor system, their hands, and they reach under and they mess everything up. Well, if you just take a thin layer of play dough or clay to put the shapes in, they can then begin to work from that. That's the only reason it's there.

In the third step we begin to move from a concrete experience to a symbolic experience by asking the parent to draw shapes in the same size as the blocks that they're working from; maybe with a square and two diamonds in a pattern. Have the child now, from seeing this pattern, reach under cover and put this together. This is a very different thing from having him work from the actual parquetry square. You see, when he sees that parquetry square or the parquetry diamond, he can always reach out there and confirm that. He knows that this is there, whether he's aware of this or not, there is a matching process going on from prior experience in handling. He cannot reach out there and pick that up, it's a symbol. I point out to the parents, this is just another symbol. They don't mean the same thing. What we're beginning to do is to bridge this information processing at a visual level between a concrete experience and a symbolic experience, and we're doing it simultaneously, in that he sees the symbol of the figure but he's matching it with a concrete experience down here. He always has his foot on the ground in that sense.

And now we reverse the system. Make a pattern under cover for him to feel and have him come up and draw the shape. Now lest you think that this is that easy, try it with some of these kids who are having problems in cracking our code, our symbol system, and you'll find that this is the level where you begin to separate the wheat from the chaff. A lot of children, although they can go from a symbol to the concrete experience and assemble the blocks, going from the concrete experience back to the symbolic to draw them gives him one heck of a time and some of them can't make it that first week at all.

Those who can, we move on to another level of symbolic experience. As we tell the parents at this point, really, there's been another symbol that we've been using for the same square and that's the sound that I've been making here, my speech, word for square and you've been hearing it. I've been hearing it too and I've been feeling it and saying it. This is another symbol. We would now ask you to give the youngster instructions as to how to place a pattern together. Let's say that's a red square that I have cocked at an angle. We'd say, "Make a pattern like this." But the child doesn't see the pattern. The child is going to hear the pattern and put a pattern together in a way with those blocks that will visually match what he's heard in terms of position and orientation and relationships in space. To tell a child how to rotate a red square 45 degrees counter-clockwise so that we'll orient this way will give you a little food for thought on how I'm going to communicate this to him with speech auditory labels so that he can visualize the thing in order to come up with it. When he gets to this point, we can drop back to a very concrete kind of language in a sense; put your hand on it like a point of door knob and turn it to the right so you have point of a square pointing right at you. It comes up with the same thing as 45 degrees counter-clockwise. You can begin to play with this then in terms of relationships of the clock, of telling time, and other things, too.

The next step is where more fun comes in, and believe me, from the information I get back from the parents, this turns out to be a lot of fun. For the first time, they've sat down and played some games with these kids as parents, where the child now tells the parent how to place these things. See this child search for the verbal labels to match a visualization that he has in his mind of what he expects to see over there, and for him to get this across to the parents so that they can visualize it to match his visualization. Or if he can't deal from the visualization, we tell them, go ahead and let him make a little pattern that he can see so he doesn't have to start with just what's in his mind, he can see it. This is the direction we would take this in.

The last step would be in reading instructions and for him to write out a set of instructions also. We tell them not to become fancy with this. Take it easy, you don't have to be fancy, it can be very simple. Take two parquetry squares, for example—and I do this with the parent. I give them a red square and a green square, and I take a red square and a green square. I say, "Put the red square on top of the green square," and usually, they put the red square down and put the green square right on top of it. I say, "Well, really what it meant was this, and I put my red square up there. They pick it up and put it up there. And I say, "Well, really what I meant was put the red square up here." Or, "Really what I meant was to put the red square here." Or, "What I really meant was to put the red square there." They get the idea quickly, put the red square on top of the green square communicates, but it communicates many possibilities. What we would like for the youngster to begin to see is this game of the possibilities of what I could visualize from what I hear. Once again, this is related to the classroom for the parent, that this is a child who may very well not hear the possibilities. It would be very much nicer if he could be a child who could raise his hand someday and ask the teacher, "Teacher, did you mean this or that?" She might very well say, "Gee, thank you, Johnny, I meant that one." But he saw some possibilities in this when he visualized those verbal instructions. He didn't get so tied up on it that it always came out just one way, never with possibilities.

So we simply fit this block around to many kinds of "on-top-of" situations. Now the parent is instructed to play this sort of thing when the child gives her instructions to go ahead and see how many possibilities the parent, from her point of view, she can make in this without saying much of anything, just letting the child watch this, to see if they begin to see what she is seeing as possibilities in what she has said. She can now run this to a more specific kind of communication.

"Auditory Span" is the next activity. This one we use very early the program, usually—maybe even the first week with many of the children. It's done with much emphasis on the visual. The first two steps as you'll read in the activity sheet simply describe repeating the digits forward and in reverse. But what the parent is instructed to do is, while doing this, observe the child to see how the child listens, what they do with their eyes while they're listening to this. And then in the 3rd step, they are asked, "Now, let's try it another way." If the child has been looking right at the parent all the time he's repeating the digits, we would say, "Now let's look over to the side," or, "let's look at the floor or the ceiling," or, "let's close your eyes," or, "let me do it behind you now." We find all kinds of differences.

In fact, about three months ago, one parent coming back at the end of a week with this and couldn't wait to spill out what she had observed with this. It was really bizarre. The child was unable all week to produce in order any more than two digits. This is forward, no less reverse. She couldn't repeat any more than two and be accurate, until she got down to the step (3-c) where it says with eyes closed. Then the mother said, "She repeated eight digits very accurately and consistently with her eyes closed." Man alive, what kind of a visual auditory world is that child trying to deal with in a classroom? No teacher is going to let that child sit there with her eyes closed so that she hears what the teacher is saying. And yet this is the way this child understands auditory information at this point. But if we can begin to expose this to the parents, to the home situation, and then through the training activities, we can begin to help these children begin to deal with that auditory visual world simultaneously. Because that's what it is anyway, it's all there together anyway. She's just internally; her own perceptual system is the one that's separating it, isolating it somehow, turning one on and another off when the other goes on. So, we begin to get at it this way, but using an auditory activity with a very definite orientation to the visual world.

This last one, "Straw Piercing" is—we use a regular drinking straw for a thing like this, unless the child can't handle it. If the child can't handle a drinking straw, we'll go to a towel tube, the cardboard holders from paper towels or toilet paper. Or you can just roll up a piece of paper and make it large enough. But let's talk about the way it starts out, where the child is asked to take pencil in each hand, look at the straw and to simultaneously move out with the pencils and pierce the ends of the straw. Initially, we do not tell him that he must just look at the center, or that he may look at the ends. We just tell him, "Pierce the ends of the straw." The only thing we ask him to do is to do it at the same time. Almost without exception, you will find the child looking from side to side. The parents will look from side to side when they try it. We let them do this. The first thing we want is the simultaneity of this. We've had adults come back on this one—as a matter of fact, one adult male said, "Doc, when I started this one this week, I thought you handed me a ringer. I didn't think you could do it. I couldn't possibly see both ends at the same time and I couldn't keep both hands moving at the same. If I couldn't see, I couldn't move. But by the middle of the week, I began to notice I could see both ends at the same time and I could move both hands at the same time. But I really thought you gave me something that was impossible for the first few days." It can be this hard.

So we tell the parent, "If it is this hard, if it's hard for the youngster, move to something larger in diameter and let him use his fingers," so he has some immediate confirmation of possibilities here, whether those possibilities are plus or minus 6 inches to start with, and let them move those plus or minus dimensions down narrower and narrower until he can begin to handle something differently. Thinking of this particular one in regard to making it relate meaningfully to other environments, we will sometimes have to sit down and talk to a teenager, particularly to make sure he is with us and not just there because it's time to be there. These guys can really move themselves if they put their minds to it, if they can be sold that this is the thing for them. This one boy I remember with this particular activity, it happened to have been assigned that week, the week I sat down and had a talk with him again by himself. I reminded him of some of the things that he enjoyed doing. For example, he liked to play football—he did play football on the high school team. He wanted to drive more than anything else. He was 16 years old and he was old enough in our state to get a learner's permit but his parents wouldn't let him near the Motor Vehicle Department. It was kind of a hassle at home constantly about whether or not he was going to get his learner's permit. They wouldn't let him go to get it because they didn't trust him behind the wheel. This guy's spatial world out here really was in miserable shape. He didn't know it/though. He also was very active in the Jr. Civil Air Patrol (CAP). He wanted to be a drill sergeant more than anything else. So I sat down and talked to him because now we had been working with him a few weeks. He couldn't handle his movement patterns with rhythm. He couldn't deal with two things at the same time visually. He couldn't listen and look at the same time. He knew he was having all these troubles on the activities but this didn't in any way mean that he related these same kinds of problems to the things he wanted to do out of the office.

So I said, "I don't care whether you play quarterback or on the line, but if you're even on the line in football and you're looking at the other guy right across from you, I'll bet you have one heck of a time hearing the signals the quarterback calls." He didn't argue with me. And I said, "As for C.A.P., you really want to be a drill sergeant there, don't you?" He said, "Yes." I said, "Don't do it, not now. Those kids will laugh you off the field. Can you imagine yourself—you know the trouble you're having in there when you hear a sound and whether your foot is in time with the sound or your hand is in time with the sound, can you imagine what's going to happen if you try to keep those kids in step with rhythm? What's going to happen to you? You're going to be out of step, they're going to be laughing all over the field." I said, "What about driving, and some of these things? You take a look this week at these activities and next week you tell me what you saw in these activities that would have any relevancy to some of these things you would want to do. You tell me what you see."

Well, it was this one of the piercing of the straw that he; again, this was one of those things where he couldn't wait to tell me. He said, "Do you know what I saw?" I said, "What did you see?" He said, "Well, it was that piercing of straw." I said, "What?" He said, "I saw two dented front fenders." And you know, we had no problems with that guy from this point on. His parents had no more problems with him about the vehicle permit. The program went along very nicely. But if we can be lucky enough sometimes to find that little thing in a relevancy between what we're doing in training and the relevancies he has in his own personal life-world outside of this office and begin to create a match here so that he knows there's a match here and it's not something done in isolation in our office, or something done in isolation at home because it's time to do the training now, we can really move these things. It's a very gratifying kind of thing. Those of you, who do spend much of your time in visual training, don't have to be told that. You know that.

There's a kind of—almost glory that you bathe in when you see these kids begin to change and you know they have a whole lifetime of change ahead of them that you've helped to establish for this child. In addition, some of the relationships begin to change in families when they begin to see these things; that this is the kind of thing that you can bathe in, too. I had a letter sent to me from a parent of a training case. This letter was sent to the optometrist who had referred the case to me and she was thoughtful enough to send me a copy of the letter that she sent to this optometrist. She said,

"Dear Dr. C: Regarding your knowledge of Lansing's perceptual problem, your concern that led us to the recommendation that Dr. J. Baxter Swartwout see him, was well-founded, and I wanted to tell you this. Also, Dr. Swartwout has seen Lansing twice, Aug. 27 and Sept. 1, and has explained the necessary optometric therapy."

I was absolutely fascinated by that. That was her—I had met the woman twice, been in the office twice. We hadn't started the training yet but she had information—she had by this time a report from me because I don't wait 6 months for a report. I have ways of doing this very simply and very easily. I have learned from other optometrists. But anyway, she had some knowledge of our language already.

"We will go ahead with it. From the bottom of my heart, I want to express our sincere appreciation to you, Dr. C., for guiding us and Lansing, in this direction. We will be in touch and no doubt Dr. Swartwout will be sending you his report on Lansing. Sincerely, thanks again."

You know, I didn't even ask this woman—and I say that because I will frequently ask my patients who have been referred by other optometrists, when we begin to see changes coming like this, I will say, "You know, we should be very grateful that Dr. X. recognized this problem and put you on the right track, especially after all the years of blind alleys that you followed. I think it would be a very nice thing if you took the time to call him and let him know that you're beginning to see the light of day with the boy's problem." I do this and I've had optometrists in our own society come up to me, beaming, that a patient of theirs had called them to thank them for making this referral. This doesn't hurt. This doesn't cost anything; and as far as this family and that mother, they're still his patients. I'm not their family optometrist. He is and they know it. I'm that boy's visual training specialist. I'm just somebody on the referring optometrists' side who is going to take care of a particular problem that he knows all about because he was the one who diagnosed it and made the referral. Don't overlook these possibilities for yourself, because not everybody has the temperament, I think, to deal with visual training. It's very trying. If your temperament is not for this, you'll try it and you won't like it. You'll try it and it won't work. But you can still have the kind of professional knowledge and ability to make the diagnosis, to pinpoint these problems, because they are optometric, they are visual, and make a referral to somebody in your own area and your own community where the work can be accomplished. And you can also bathe in the same kind of reflected glory that, I'll tell you, you feel from these parents. It's a real thing.

Lecture V

This topic is "A 5-Point Philosophy for Visual Training." Some of you might think that's all I do, is visual training. I don't. I sat down a few months back to try to pull together some of these things you find yourself going in 10 different directions at the same time and find yourself changing your point of view and your whole approach to training. I've gone through a fantastic metamorphosis in terms of the training that's being done in my office. I started out 21 years ago doing visual training. I think I was working with training cases before I had my first private examination, literally. I went into a partnership practice and my partner, in his wisdom of several years of practice ahead of me, knew I was going to be a dead weight around the place for a while, so he had saved up a lot of training cases. I was dumped in like the infant in the swimming pool to learn how to swim, and I learned something about visual training from the interaction of these patients. But it was nothing like the visual training that we're doing now. It has grown, it has changed. I've worked with groups of 6 and 8 and 10. I've kept all of the parents out in the reception area. I let them drop them off from their car and let them come on in and we'd work, to the point where the way we are working now it's kind of a family affair.

But this family affair business really comes into view in this first point of this approach to the philosophy that I think I have for visual training. I might state it this way; that I would like to establish a self-fulfilling prophecy for success early in any training program that I'm going to have anything to do with. One of those ways is to get the family involved in it on a level of understanding of what they're involved in. That's one of the reasons I want both parents there. That way if there are questions, we can find out about these aspects of them early. This helps us anticipate if there are going to be difficulties; let's know about them early rather than later. And this helps us to give the parents enough information.

One of the other things that came out of this little study group meeting up here is that I do use a report form. I got this report form from the office of Drs. Keith Wilson and William Nelson in Chula Vista.[8] It's based on the Educator's Guide and Checklist, essentially, and it has saved me untold hours of report-making and has given me untold value in public relations. As an illustration, I had a phone call about 6 months ago from a Sister at the College of St. Rose in Albany asking me if I would speak to her graduate students in the psychophysiology of perception and reading problems. I had done this for other teachers at St. Rose, normally every year, but this one was a new one. It seems she had gotten from one of her students one of my report forms all filled out, one of her students is a teacher in a school system some miles south of us. We had just started to work with a little boy in her class. She thought it would be great if I could come down and talk about the information that was on this report form. We decided we would work right from that particular case, simply blanked out names and so on, copied the thing for all of the students in the class, who were educators from a very wide surrounding area, some administrative levels, most of them in remedial or developmental reading teaching, and some of them classroom teachers, working towards a degree. But, little things like this can happen from it. It does communicate rather well. I'm sorry, perhaps I should have—as long as I'm talking about it, I didn't plan to talk about it, but it kind of came up here and it fits into this, because it's part of the establishing prophecy for success. We can then begin to work from a common basis and knowledge, even to the language, such as you've heard in this letter that I read. It's just a little thing but she knows the difference between optometric training, I think, and the educational visual training that might be done in a classroom. It's a very different thing.

One of the other things about this prophecy is that it has two sides, as so many things do. An illustration here is, I think, in order. I'm

---

8. *Editor's note: This is the practice that Dr. Robert Wold eventually took over and from which he served COVD over many years.*

thinking of a 14-year-old youngster who had just moved on into his Jr. High school in a rather small community some miles north of us where everybody knows everybody else. This was a boy whose reputation had preceded him from his grammar school to the Jr. High. Before he ever even got there—the year before he was to arrive, the teachers were already buzzing about the fact that he was going to be there next year. Oh, boy! One of his teachers that year had been a next-door neighbor of his, so she was certainly very able to confirm all of the suspicions and maybe add a few new ones that the other teachers might have had about this fellow coming up. Now he wasn't a bad kid, he wasn't a delinquent; he wasn't in trouble in that way. He just wasn't learning much. He was constantly doing the wrong thing at the wrong time; he was a behavioral disorder problem in the classroom. But, once we got him in visual training things began to move with this guy real well. I was very happy about this, the mother was very happy about this. By the time we had finished 2 ½ months or 3 months of training whatever it was, it was about time for a report card to come through. It came in with this thing, no change. Well, it was kind of early and you don't expect an awful lot at that stage.

The progress evaluation came up after another two or three months and in time again for another report card, anyway—no change. Well, I was a little upset at this because from all that I could see and measure, if there's any reliability in what we're doing, there was change in this boy in terms of visual information processing, in terms of being able to deal with information at a visual level, and there was no change in any of these areas of performance. This child had originally been referred by the school psychologist which made this next step a little bit easier, because we already had a speaking relationship. I called the man and asked him about the boy. He said, "Interesting that you should call now." He had just done some testing on him and he said, "What you are telling me, I see in my testing, too. That's strange he's not doing any better." I said, "Have you discussed any of this with the teachers?" He said, "No. I did speak to them early in the school year after I made the referral of the boy to you." I said, "I wonder if you'd mind contacting them again, seeing what's going on, seeing if there is something happening that we don't know about?" He said, "Not a bit. I'll do that." He called me back a few days later and said that he had contacted each of the teachers. What we had going for us was the most beautiful self-fulfilling prophecy for failure that I've ever seen. Those teachers had seen nothing in that boy that they had ever seen in that boy before. He sat in the same corner way in the back of the room, isolated, talked around, put to the side, and he was producing and doing nothing different than he had done before. He hadn't even had an opportunity to show them. I don't know how the situation could have been so successful in such a negative way, but it was.

And it turned out within the next few months, around came another marking period, but now he was just as successful in the positive way as soon as the teachers saw the results the psychologist had to show them from the testing, which had shown that now the boy was able to learn. They were suddenly able to teach him. This is really no different from the experiment that I read about. I think the study may have been done here in a school system where the classrooms were twinned in a school system. The teacher was approached in one by the experimenters. "We almost apologize to you for the problems you're going- to have this year. It won't be held against you no matter what happens to these kids. No matter how many of them fail or whatever happens, these kids are just not going to learn. It's a bad bunch and we really feel sorry for you." It was this sort of approach. The other teacher in the other school with the twinned group was approached: "Oh, we'd love to be in your shoes this year. You're going to have a great time with these children. They are just so ready. All of the tests we've done, all the indications we have indicate that they're just going to be a beautiful group for you to work with this year. They're going to learn like crazy." They did, and the other group didn't. This self-fulfilling prophecy is very potent. If we can't have sufficient confidence in our own tools, in our own tests to let us know how this youngster is performing or capable of performing, we can have things like this upsetting our applecart and proving to us that we had failed when we actually had had a beautiful success. It may still be a total failure.

It's a very serious thing to think about, and until the time is reached that we have better communication with other disciplines, this is something that any optometrist doing visual training, especially dealing with children with learning disabilities had better take into account. Keep some kind of contact, some kind of communication channel open in the schools where this may happen. You know that even laboratory animals will respond to this sort of attitude on the part of the trainer, from what I hear? Some of the men, in psychology, who work with rats, do this training of rats, and you have to be careful what technician you put on your rats or you're going to louse up your experiment. The rats know a technician who loves them and then they perform better for them. Love is very important in our office. We love one another and we love those parents and we love those kids. We let those parents know that we think so much of them for having taken on this kind of a responsibility—and if you realize what a responsibility it is for those parents, and some of those parents know this, oh, boy, they figure this out fast. If you don't bring it up yourself, you'll have some of them bringing it up to you. "Do you think I'm capable of doing this, Dr.?" I mean, after all, the school system has failed for how many years? The tender, loving care that they've had from other specialists and other disciplines has failed for so many years. How can we expect then that the parent is going suddenly to become successful? We have to have a very strong position to work from, and we let the parent know that we appreciate their willingness to do this. And that last day in the office when they come in—some of those parents won't even tell the kids it's going to be the last day until they're on their way from home, because they're afraid the kids are going to be too upset.

We like to see them running into the office and have to push them out. We do. It's a horrible job sometimes to get one family cleared out of the training area so that anther one can get in there. Because at that last split second, all the other little kids who have been so nice to stay out in the front reception area for a while, they know it's over, they come on in, 5, 6, 7 of them, all around the place and they've got to handle a few things before you can get them out so the next group can come in. It's hard. If they can enjoy this, they can enjoy learning.

But there's more to it than simply recognizing that we may have some mismatches in these other environments and among other disciplines. It still is a matter of programming our own procedures at levels with which the child can achieve. And yet at the same time, explore this thing well enough to find out what he can't achieve in such a way that he won't take it as another personal affront and another demonstration and confirmation of has tremendous ability to fail. This is one of the things that these kids have done most successfully and most consistently up to this point. They have failed to be able to stand up to the level of performance expected of them in many environments; at school, at home, and with their peers. This matter of helping him to be willing enough to explore some things, to challenge him enough and yet not frustrate him, and keep him going is part of this success prophecy.

One of the things we find helpful in this is this business of taking the activities away at the end of the week. Supposing at the end of the week, the parent says, "Gee, he had trouble with this one. This one he really didn't do very well with." We'll have parents say then, "Maybe we should do this one again this week." I say, "Oh, no, especially we don't want him to do that one again this week." I can normally, usually point out one of the particular activities that I've already selected for this coming week and say, "Look, there are attributes of that particular activity he had trouble with in this one that he'll be doing this week. Let's take a piece of it. Let's not put him on the same thing he's told us in a week's time, I don't handle well, I can't understand easily, I'm having trouble with, it distresses me, I tighten up on it and I'm not going to learn well on it. "Get rid of it." We'll go back to it in 3 months as we do, and 9 times out of 10, that little guy is going to be able to handle that thing and those parents come back for the progress evaluation after this and they say, "It's just amazing. He didn't practice it. We haven't done that for 3 months and he couldn't even do it the week we left it 3 months ago. Now he can do it." And I say, "Great, he's learned to put some pieces together inside. He begins to know how to problem-solve and relate to situations outside on the basis of a different understanding of his own level of skills, his own organization." This is what we're looking for.

On the other hand, there is the parent who comes in at the end of the week and says, "Look at the progress he made on this one. You can just see it going up like this. Boy, we'll do that one again for another week and it will be even better, right?" And I say, "Wrong." Why? It is because I'm not interested in making him into a virtuoso on any one of these procedures or techniques. I'm only interested in having him explore some relationships that we can establish within that procedure, broaden the base of organization, see some relationships between it and some other activities that he's done, including the one that he had trouble with. And in another week, also including this and the one he had trouble with, because this is what I think makes the difference at the end of three months. He goes back to see this one again that he couldn't do. Now he has all these relationships he's been growing and seeing and understudying, and puts the pieces together differently. So the activities, the parents are told, are used for one purpose only; to give him an opportunity to explore some of his own potentials, to develop a broader base with which to still be able to handle this activity. This is all part of the programming that leads towards the establishment of a self-fulfilling prophecy for success.

This would be true, I guess, in any curriculum planning. If you have a good curriculum that will meet the needs of the levels of the individuals within it, it's going to be a more successful curriculum. Then when you get the presenter of the curriculum, the parent in this case, our staff in the office including myself, so that there's confidence in what they're doing, those assistants, they just know that there's going to be a success in any new case that we start. We get a little itchy sometimes. We'd like to move it along faster, and we'll sometimes tell the patient, the parents too, "Gee, we'd almost like to wish away the next 2 or 3 months, but I guess we'll have to wait because we think there's going to be so much change here." We're not afraid to make some predictions that we're going to move towards success, because I think we're working from a very strong, solid position in making that prediction. It's been too many times confirmed and it's been too few times denied; our observations. I can speak very positively about it because I've had 21 years of doing it. I don't think anyone starting out in it immediately is going to have this confidence in what they're doing. You have to develop this and build it, but there's no place you can start up here if you're down here. You move. You change, you learn. The potential in visual training is so great that it would be pretty hard not to succeed, I think.

The second thing that I've kind of pulled out of, formed something of a philosophy of this is to: direct the training towards opportunity to predict and monitor process. This goes along with the comment

I made that the procedures are assigned, not with the idea in mind that the child should become a virtuoso in performing this particular activity, but rather to see what we can help him with in discovering things about himself that he somehow, up to this point, has not learned; that he can learn how to look and listen at the same time. Take the ball on the string, for example. To hear the hand on the ball and the foot on the floor and to still see it going in a straight line and still know he's touched it gently. To have heard this contact of hand and foot and the simultaneity of it, to have felt the foot and the hand and the simultaneity of that, and at the same time perhaps have him count with and recognize that his voice is coming out predictive to his visual pattern, that it comes out as a 1, not as a 1,[9] and for him to hear the difference in that. Because one is a tactual prediction and the other is a visual prediction, and I'll bet half of you here didn't hear or see the difference. I just gave you a tactual prediction that sounded like a visual prediction, and it wasn't. This is the way this child operates. But you can see it and the parents can begin to see it. You'll read it in the activity sheet.

The really important thing is to get him to discover things about himself. In this way, he's going to be able to put some pieces together a little differently, in ways he hasn't been able to deal with before. Another way of thinking about this is to think in terms of relationships that he's going to be able to see, more relationships at any one time. He's going to be able to take a bigger volume of space in visually at any one time. And at the same time, deal with other relationships that are ongoing.

The third step in this would be to direct the practice in optometric training towards the ability to maintain the central task against distraction. This is the opposite point of view of the cubicle, for example. Those of you who remember reading Gerald N. Getman's chapters,[10] maybe three years ago, where he described what they finally decided their approach to the cubicle was. It was to help the child get back into the usual environment, because this is where

---

9. *The differences Dr. Swartwout made with his voice are hard to capture in print. One of these would have been said easily and clearly and the other loudly and with poor timing.*

10. *Dr. G.N. Getman wrote a number of chapters for the OEP. His book, "Developmental Optometry," is available from OEP through the on line store at www.oepf.org. In addition he wrote: "Vision, Audition and Problems of Learning" OEP Curriculum II Series, 1968-69.*

he had to be. Eventually, this is where he has to be. They moved him gradually away from looking at the back wall of the cubicle to looking at one of the other sidewalls, and then to the other sidewall, and then moving him out a little bit so he had maybe just a little bit of the space around him, and add a little bit more, until he could begin to deal with the other life style situations that go on all around him. The other sounds, the other visual areas. This is what we do with our training. In the office, we expose the parents to this concept, that we want him to be able to deal with the task that he'd been put on, and at the same time to be able to deal with other things. The parents get examples of it. They have to have reinforcement constantly because they see it for the specific item you're talking about now but they don't necessarily relate it to the setting of the table from the other side, the way that father did immediately. This relates to the business of looking at the tack and noticing the string without losing fixation on the tack, this sort of thing. Piercing a ring from over here and when we say, "Now I want you to be aware of your hand over here," after we have already said, "Keep looking at the ring out here, but feel your hand over here," and they still do this. It's the simultaneity of being able to deal with these distractions.

This was a distraction. They were asked to look here. That's the visual. "Look there; match it with what you feel here while you are looking there." On an activity of this sort, you'll find the child who has been missing all over the place. Once he begins to feel something at the same time he's seeing something, and not see this and then see that and then see that and then see this and try to put the two together; you know it as it changes, where they were missing it now they begin to hit it. They begin to put some relationships in it. But this is also distraction.

Did I mention the controlled reader to you as a group? One of the best examples of it with the adults and the children, both, are on the controlled reader which we use. With both children and adults this is a visual task. We have the patient reading as it goes.

Use anywhere from one to two grade levels below his reading level. The best we can establish what his reading level is, we drop it down, if we can, one or two grade levels below that, because we're not interested in teaching reading. All I want him on is something he can handle visually, a highly central task, and at the same time, I want to know if he knows what he has read. But while he's reading, we're putting lenses in for accommodative rock and asking him questions about size, space, relationships, and any other changes he might see. We're dropping prisms in, or rotary prisms, moving it and asking about spatial relationship changes. We have a red and a green lens in the phorometer also. We're asking him about the color—does it change? What color is it now? And so on. And at the end of this, he's then asked questions about what he read.

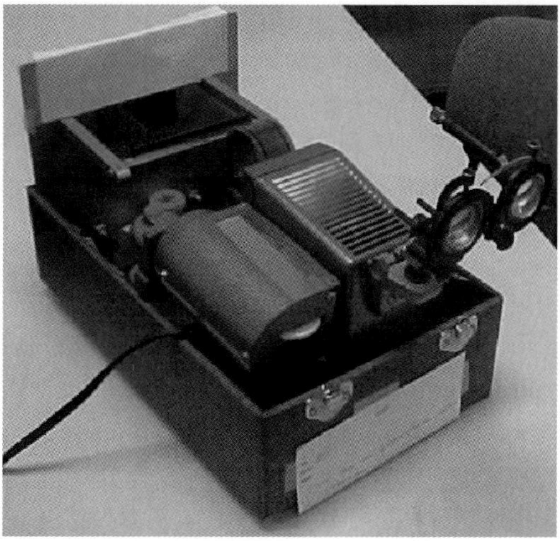

Figure 2: Controlled Reader with prism head attached. The Controlled Reader was a product of Educational Developmental Laboratories (EDL) of Huntington, NY but is not made as of this writing. An excellent substitute for the guided reading with graded stories at controlled speeds is VisionBuilder ™ which can be purchased from OEP.

All the time he's been listening to us, all the time he's been giving us other answers, other responses of having seen these other visual phenomena, simultaneously while he's reading. Do you know what we get with these kids after the first week or two of this? We don't usually put this in with most of them until about the 4th week. Maybe 50% correct on the comprehension test, and quickly within the next week or so it rises up to 70%, and we try to maintain it, hold it pretty much around 70%. If they start getting up to 80% and 90% on the thing, I have to talk to the assistants, because they don't like to push the speed up too much. The goal of this isn't speed on this. That's not the push. However that is one additional push once they get to be good enough, Then I want to move, I don't want them to sit in one spot at any time on these things. So we push for speed as long as they're able to maintain some kind of percentage of comprehension.

We did this with our study group also. With the study group one night, each man had a turn at this. And you know, the assistants insisted that they come to that study group meeting. This is a technique that they handle in the office. They wouldn't have missed that for the world because they were making all kinds of conjectures, between themselves as to what they were going to find with the optometrists when they put them on this task and began talking to them while they were reading and then ask questions about what they read. We had seen adults in the office when we put them on this just about ready to pick up the whole instrument, table and everything, and heave it at the assistant. I've heard voices raised in the training room; one male voice, I'll never forget it. "Do you want me to read or do you want me to listen to you?" This is the kind of reaction you get with many of these training cases.

With the optometrists, I think they were a little nasty, I really don't know, but I think the assistants were just a little bit nasty with the study group, because not one of those guys was able to get anything more than 10% comprehension. That was on 6th grade material. We didn't even include the Jr. High school material. Seriously, that's what happened. But seriously, this is the kind of an environment, the kind of a situation that we all find ourselves in. How many of you can study, how many of you can sit down and read while there are other things going on around you? How many of the kids can do it? This is a problem with them; the auditory world out there, the world of sound doesn't stop because the child is sitting in the classroom to read, unless he stops it from within. If he stops it from within, this is a perceptual constriction as far as I can see and it means he has fewer bits of experience available to him to deal with the decoding of those symbols. That's the way I look at it. So if he can deal with these potentials, sort it out in the periphery, the things that don't relate, they don't relate. They're immaterial at the moment, but they're not going to interfere, so we orient any of the training activities to move them in this direction. Let's take another one over here. Before I leave that, though, there's kind of a key word and I've used it many times—that's *simultaneity*, just as we've used *relationships;* more relationships with simultaneity, a big volume. Vision is not a plane, like the page. Vision is still a volume, even when we read, unless we do something about it inside on a perceptual level again and constrict.

The fourth item on this is to direct the optometric training towards the meaningful life experiences of the patient. I've given illustrations of this sort of thing already. The boy who came in with the two dented front fenders. We know something of the child's hobbies or we know something of the dissatisfaction he has with himself, the poor feeling of worthiness that he may feel for himself. On a case like this, as soon as we can begin to see some little things change; for example the parents may begin to report these changes, or sometimes it is a paper that comes home from school for the first time in this child's life with a nice comment on it by the teacher. Or without its being all marked up or with its having a passing grade on it or something like that. We'll ask these kids, how do you feel now? Did it make you feel good? So that we can help them move on towards being aware that this is part of their feeling, that this is part of their reason for doing these things. We try to relate the improvement in the hand writing, or the organization on the paper, or whatever the parents—because they tell us what the changes are and they'll usually bring in other things and say, "This is what it was like." We relate these things for the parents and then also, to be sure that they see the relationship, which they probably have but it helps to say it again, the things that they've been doing at home that would do this. The kinds of arm movement activities at the chalkboard that we've already told them about that we are interested in because we want the child to hold the chalk in his hand so he can begin to move the wrist.

So now the first articulation is here. Week after week he's doing something to articulate differently, to move the ball differently as you'll see in the ball-on-string phase to where we'll even have him controlling it this way in a rotation. But get these movement patterns that are visually predictive. It's interesting the number of times one of the first things we begin to see that are reportable, that we can relate to the child to help him feel better about himself, is the handwriting, the organization of the things on the paper.

The other thing that would relate in this area of helping to move the training towards meaningful experiences is to avoid something. Part of the difficulty or problem, I think, we run into in training is that we do take an attitude sometimes that this guy cannot make Harmon circles, let's say, so we're going to teach him to make these circles, and so on. And do them in the other directions. We had an experience where this was the specific situation. We were seeing a youngster who had been in training some three to 4 months prior to my seeing him, traveling a number of miles for this and eventually being referred for continuation of the training to my office. Our testing indicated that he must have been very far down on the totem pole when he started that training a few months ago, because he still had a lot of problems, so we started him off pretty much as we would have almost any child. This boy was in his very early teens, maybe 12 or 13. We got to this activity, because we had done a little quick test on this particular one anyway, Harmon circles—that it didn't look good at all on the test the assistants did, so I assigned it for one week. At that point, the mother said—she hadn't said anything about it before, but at that point she said, "Oh, he won't have any problem with that one. We worked on that for 3 months until he got it." What had happened was just this sort of thing; that he wasn't able to do this and it became the goal of the optometrist doing the training for the child to be able to do that activity. This in no way states that this was a goal for the child at all. This was something he had to get done to get a monkey off his back, and he learned to do it after 3 months to the satisfaction of the optometrist and the parents. The mother observed these sessions, incidentally, and she said that to her satisfaction, he could do it. You know, we sent him to the chalkboard to do this again that day of the training and he still couldn't do it.

I don't know what kind of habituation this is that we can learn to do something to pass the test now and zing, down it goes. But, it reminds me an awful lot of the kind of studying that children will do to pass the spelling test tomorrow. If they do have a long enough memory span to hold over until tomorrow and pass it, then right after it, they've forgotten it. I can remember taking examinations like this going through school, going through college I can remember taking exams like this. Out of sight, out of mind. I passed it now, forget it, it's not going to relate to anything I'm going to do. But this kind of learning to be done therapeutically, I think defeats our purpose. We're not establishing goals that are meaningful to the child. They somehow are meaningful to us. We want to train a saccadic; we want to train a fixation, we want to train pursuit, we want to train accommodation, and so on. I only want to work with accommodation and saccades and pursuits against this broader frame of reference of the child doing other things simultaneously; seeing other relationships at the same time; being able to listen at the same time he's doing his accommodative rock; being able to use his hands at the same time that he's doing accommodative rock; being able to listen to a metronome and rock back and forth while he's doing accommodative rock. You know we find some kids who can't clear in accommodative rock until the metronome is put on? And then they can clear? If they can do it against rhythm, an auditory rhythm, that's a good thing.

But these are some of the things you begin to learn about vision when you begin to see to it that these other things are plugged in simultaneously and that we don't just train our skills in isolation but relate it to a broader spectrum and, hopefully, towards a direction that will relate to the child's other worlds.

The fifth thing on this is to maintain my own awareness of the role of vision in the techniques and procedures used, This is very important. Over the years, I've run across from time to time some very lost optometrists, some very confused optometrists who perhaps have become enamored of things that they've heard about other disciplines and what other professions are doing and other techniques and approaches to these problems, and they step right off the deep end to do someone else's thing without having the base to do that thing from. We have within our own discipline a good, solid grounding in physiology, as good as any profession. On top of that, being a remedial profession, we have a basis that other professions who can test some of these situations and come up with very interesting diagnoses would love to have the base in physiology in order to do something about It. Or, other remedial professions who don't have the base in physiology to look really at the underlying systems that may cause the difficulty in the higher level performance, such as reading, such as with the asymmetries in the visual system that we can measure, the effects of lenses on the input side of the system that can alter the whole output system. This is within our frame of reference to recognize.

But this doesn't by any means mean that we cannot or should not utilize information from other disciplines, any more than other disciplines should not utilize information from ours. From our own point of view, we would use it. I think maybe an example of this is auditory span. I'm quick to point out to the parents when I assign a thing like this, this looks as though we're going to start doing some listening training. Maybe I am, but at the same time—I don't say maybe I am to the parent. I say, "What I'm interested in is, that I want him to be able to do some visual things at the same time that he's listening." I point out that the visual is involved in the activity. I've had many interesting experiences in meeting people with backgrounds and training and education that I would never had suspected they have. And if I had been careless enough to try to use the tools of another discipline in an ape-like way of simply mimicking the way it's used in other disciplines, I could have found myself in a lot of hot water. I don't know how many of you feel that you've seen potential for this kind of thing. But I have parents who have much better grounding than I'll ever have in clinical psychology, in reading training, developmental—the whole background of development. I have some training aspects of it as it relates to the visual, but some of these people have training in many other areas. We have some patients who are physical education developmental specialists—the aspect discussed yesterday. These people can tell me something about these things. So when I use physical movement organization in visual training, I want that grounded firmly in my own thinking and in my own mind that it's visually related that I'm interested in. Then I can demonstrate to myself and to that individual, no matter how much he knows about physical education and development, that when he bends over perhaps and gets into a warped or twisted position and he can see a suppression occur, he knows that we're both talking the same language, we're both talking the same integrations, we're both talking the same kind of language in helping a child, but from other points of view. I'm no longer stepping on his toes and he's no longer stepping on mine. But it's so easy, I think, to find yourself in a situation where you begin to talk as a psychologist perhaps when you should be talking as an optometrist.

Let's have some questions now:

MEMBER: Do you spend "x"[11] hours a week in the training program?

---

11. *Editor's Note: In correspondence with Dr. Swartwout in June of 2010 he recalls the question being asked in an open ended manner such that the "x" is appropriate here. He asked his families to attempt to get 30-minutes of home therapy done on the days they were not in the office. During the home phase of vision therapy this totaled 3.5*

DR. SWARTWOUT: With an individual case. I spend so many hours a week with an individual case in a training program, right.

MEMBER: Is the amount of time spent in training in the office and at home a factor in the success of the case, as well as the particular techniques that are used?

DR. SWARTWOUT: Yes. Again, in conversation something came up. A parent last week called, two days before their scheduled office visit. The mother was just—you could just hear her. She's a very tight, tense individual anyway, she has lots of problems, and she's had lots of things in her young life as it is; enough to tighten anybody up. She has several little kids. She called up and said, "Dr. Swartwout, I haven't been able to get at the training much this week; only once or twice." The telephone I had almost felt like it was being squeezed from the other end. She said, "I think we'd better call this off." I said, "All right." There was a silence on the other end and she said, "How much time is necessary to work in?" I said, "Well, that kind of depends." She said, "What am I going to have to do when we finish the program? Is it going to be all finished then?" I'd gone over all this with her, she knew all the answers to this but she'd forgotten them. She really didn't want to quit the program, apparently. Anyway, I talked to her a little bit more and there was some screeching and screaming at the other end of the line and she said, "Get out of here." Well, the kids had come in. She was really—oh, I don't know what happened to her that day. She said, "I'm too busy. I have so many things--" and she went down a list of things. I said, "How much time can you spend?" She said, "Well, I don't find too much trouble with maybe 3 or 4 days a week." And she said, "Besides, is it going to be all over at 10 weeks?" I said, "Remember what we talked about, that the whole orientation of the program is to put information in your hands so that you can go at your pace and the child's pace to begin to resolve the problem." This is what we tell them. We're not about to solve a visual problem in 10 weeks. They have to put it to use over a period time. The outcome of this was that she came in Friday for her appointment and she's all calm again about the training because she's got some things ordered—that we're not going to crowd her and we're not going to crowd the child and give it enough time. I'll still be able to do the job for them, but

<u>hours of vision therapy per week if no practice were ever missed. There was a sense of flexibility and realism knowing that some days the home practice would not be done.</u>

it won't come through at the same rate, but she's well aware of this at this point.

MEMBER: How many comments do you get from parents about the side effects or benefits that they receive in going through this training?

DR. SWARTWOUT: It's a very interesting thing. Some of the parents are completely unaware that they are in a training session, that they're going through a tremendous amount of training themselves. I remember one young couple that came in with an autistic child that we did some training with. These two people—they were real angels with this boy. He was 12 and he was very much of a problem. The only thing he had on his mind was trains. He'd break into almost anything to talk about trains and the wheels going around and the smoke and so on. But we were able to help them. One of the things we found with the parents was, here the boy was working over there and I'd say something to them and they'd hear something over there, they'd be over there and I'd be cut out. Then I'd say something that got their attention and they'd be over here and they'd be cut out. This was the most difficult thing for these two parents, to deal with what was going on over there and what was going on here simultaneously. They got training in simultaneity and in relationships and in visual and auditory space organization while they sat at the desk with me, while the training was going on. But it took weeks for them to be able to sit there comfortably. We talked about it. You could see that it was hard for them. I told them then, "This is going to be rather difficult for you." It was obvious, you know, but I want to get it out, I want them to be aware of it. "It's going to be difficult for you because I want you to be aware. I want you to keep one eye and ear over there and one eye and one ear over here." Not literally, you know.

Even with these parents, you could see why with this boy. They were very concerned about him. He could get himself into all kinds of trouble in no time flat in the office, but the assistant, we've worked with kids like this before and we were able to help him. But I think we helped them in helping them to help him through this kind of a training situation that they were in without even realizing it at first as a training situation.

MEMBER: Do you think the teenager or any training case or any patient or any individual who can deal with music on, read, eat, do a number of other things all at the same time, and maybe even studying, is in a better position to cope with life situations, and make better students and generally make out better in general situations?

DR. SWARTWOUT: I would think so. Now I'm not saying that he at that time is using himself most effectively in his studying, but I think he has the potential for it. As I think of some of these youngsters that we see where the individual is so stressed that one college student who would study in the last room in the house. This was one of these double-deckers, deep narrow homes, must have been five or six rooms deep and he was way at the end of the house, way in the back. He had a younger brother who would come in from school, while he was studying in this room six rooms back, who would close the door and this guy would have a tantrum out in the room, six rooms back. The was a college boy.

Or the brother would come in and maybe he'd remember to close the door softly and forget and turn the radio on, or TV on or something. This would trigger another tantrum out in the back, six rooms deep. When that boy studied, nobody could talk above a whisper in the house. He flunked out of college. We didn't get to him in time. He was so stressed, so tight, so tense. That boy, if he was looking at something, he couldn't hear—If he was still seeing what he was looking at. He was so tense in his visual and his motor areas that just to demonstrate for himself, so he could see for himself, the stresses that are related to mind and body; we had him do a preschool activity on the chalkboard tracing a circle template. And now we said, "Put it over here on the side and trace it." You know, he couldn't keep the chalk against the template. He couldn't handle anything unless it was on center.

I'm concerned about this thing and I perhaps should have said more about it because it does relate to this business of dealing with relationships and dealing with information simultaneously, that under conditions of stress, the individual will tend to constrict and tighten up. Not just in his perceptual fields as V.I. Shipman[12] has stated that

---

12. *This quote was often used by A.M. Skeffington. Skeffington heard it read before the Eastern Psychological Association, Philadelphia, 1955: " Stress brings up a constriction of the perceptual fields, and the child observes less, sees less, remembers less, learns less, and becomes generally less efficient."*

Skeffington keeps referring to that's so meaningful, but his body will tighten up. The movement pattern stress. This is no time to sit down and problem solve or read. By the same token, parents or children or the student who is under mental stress is in no position to sit down and do a lot of this. He also will tend to tighten up. It's a mind and body relationship. Tighten the body, the mind tightens. Or, tighten the mind and the body tightens, or the perceptual worlds or however you want to describe it. But I still see this in a visual sense. That the movement patterns of the eyes are a part of the movement patterns of the general movement pattern system—motor. The sensory aspect of the visual system, the information processing, the symbol decoding, the intersensory organizations in visual space, this is part of that minding system. I have the two systems simultaneously involved in any visual act. If I tighten this on the general motor level, I can't help but see it's going to affect the visual motor level. And from the general motor level into the mind level into the information processing level. That's why I answered the question the way I did. I would say, he's probably in better shape from my point of view.

Lecture VI

This is something that kind of came up rather late in the planning of my part in this program—this bridging the gap between the training room and the classroom. There are a number of very specific things that I do at the very last training visit with the parent to further this notion that what we're doing in visual training is not something to be considered in isolation by the parent or by the child in particular. It's something we would like to have the child, in particular, recognize as a part of his general daily kind of living routines. It seems, at least from my experience in working with visual training cases that many times they know that visual training's going to be done during the day. That's kind of a bamboo or iron curtain segment, they go into the training in the office or the home, the training is over and forgotten and they go on about their business. It just simply means that if we can help them to be aware of some of the concepts—not the procedures but the concepts and see relationships between the things that they do in the classroom or at play, we seem to be getting faster results; the more we can communicate this idea to the parents. One of the things that I do all throughout the training, visits with the parents, is to point this kind of possibility of drawing relationships between activities from one week to the next, between activities during the week, between activities or the demands for performance or skill on various procedures with ball-playing, with copying from board to desk, and so on. We've laid the groundwork for some sort of awareness for developing a broad-based idea of relationships, in other words.

On this last visit, among other things that are a little bit different are usually three to four specific additional assignments that they have not had before. Now up to this point, the training session has been just the same as any of the others. They've gotten a new set of activities to do for that final 10th week at home. The youngster has gone through some additional training in the office. One difference is that we have done some additional testing on this last visit for comparative purposes. I alluded to this yesterday when I described the Van Orden star and how we used it on the 10th session in most of the cases to help the parent realize that the child has now gained some difference in point of view or ability to deal with information more symmetrically between the two visual systems. There are other tests we re-do depending on the individual, so we point this out to the parent, too.

The second thing we do is, with these 3, 4, or 5 it might be particularly different activities, we mark them differently, talk about them differently and we say, "Do your 10th week activities just as you've been doing the 1st, the 2nd, the 9th and so on. But with these that I'm going to be describing to you, I want you to wait until you've finished your 10th week and to then go back to the first week's activities again, re-do those; recognizing the child is going to be refining what he has already learned to do about these. He's going to be seeing it differently. Look for differences. You have, as a parent now, built in continuing testing training program, and when we see you in 2 months for a progress evaluation, I'll be interested in your observations of how your child went back to activities that perhaps he was unable to do well at all when we left them, and now without having practiced on them is perhaps able to do them better. Then on the 11th week as you do these activities that were already assigned, I want you to take one of these -- and we'll go over them one at a time with them -- and on the 1st day of that 11th week, do one of these. On the 2nd day, do another one, on the 3rd day you do still another, and round-robin these right on through that week and the following week and the following weeks. These activities are little different from most of the activities that you've been doing at home," I tell them. They are specifically more oriented to a classroom type situation, the kinds of demands that the child should recognize as reminding him of school.

Now this is done not in school but right at home so that there is this kind of a reminder of a classroom type orientation during the course of the visual training practice at home. And we want the parents to recognize this, that's why we tell them. And we want the parents to have the child recognize this. So they tell the child. There is this kind of awareness; there is this on-going relatedness between the training and the classroom. They're even talking about it. Let's go through these—there are several of them in the new sheets that were passed out this morning. Normally, I do not assign all of these that you have in hand to any one particular patient. If we do want them eventually to have all these things, we'll wait until perhaps the progress evaluation in two months and then add some others as we reduce the number of these additional items that they're working with. As far as the control and management of this kind of thing is concerned, remembering that the parents already have 5 activities that they're going to be doing on that 11th week—and here is another activity that is going to take time, and I don't want them to spend more time on this—we advise those people to work for 30 minutes a day. Not that there's anything magic about 30 minutes, but in general it seems to be a segment of time that the parents can find and a segment of time that a child will abide by. It's not that much of a demand on him and it seems to produce some of the results that you're looking for. It just seems to work out this way. So we tell them, "Don't increase your time. You're adding another activity. You may spend up to 10 minutes on these particular activities, so if you only get 2 or 3 of the original activities done, fine. The following day, do the other 2 or 3, but the next day, you do still another of these special item activities." So that they will rearrange, perhaps, the way they've been handling their time, but not increase the time.

The first of these is Flash Card. This is pointed out as a continuation of some activities that we've been doing in the office with the child on tachistoscope. The parent has observed the child in performance on the LL series, the XVA and the P [13] series at least to some degree, because we explore this. If we don't have time to do a lot of training on it, we explore it, normally, right from the 1st week. We don't wait on the tach until other changes occur; we start this right out in the first week. When I show them on this particular sheet that you have on top that says "Flash Card" that what they are to do is to make up a series of 3 x 5 cards and put these designs on them. If you'll look at the upper left under examples, there's a square and a triangle. As we look at these, I point to them and I say, "If you'll notice on these first two, you have two shapes the same size, but different shapes. The next two are two shapes, the same shape but different sizes. And the next two are the same size and shape but they are different position in space, different orientations. This is what I would like you to do at home. Use these concepts to make up a series of 3 x 5 cards to put some likes and differences on for him to explore on a flash basis." And we tell the parent to say, "Ready now," quick like this just flash and expose and the child is asked then to reproduce it on paper. Of course they've seen them do this with the work in the office on the chalkboard so it's not that new to them.

The next two that you see to the right of those, I point out, "You can make up another series of cards that would have similar shapes, similar arrangements, but put some figure ground relationships in them. Some might have dots in them, shaded areas, blacked out areas, curlicue tails, or what have you, but they have some little differences within the general geometric shape that is utilized." By this time I tell them, too, that normally as a starting point, five cards would be enough on any one particular set, because with five 3 x 5 cards with utilizing these ideas, they actually have 20 different exposures; right side up, upside down, and on end, and reverse it back. So they have a number of ways of dealing with it. I tell them that really, what we're after, however, comes down in step 24 which you'll read. "As performance improves, find new ways to use this activity." Then it goes on to give some examples of what we mean by this. And I say, "Now you've noticed that there are some tic-tac-toe designs and some arrows. What we mean by that is something

---

13. These are part of the Lyons and Lyons series of training visualization and visual imagery. The book, "Visualization, Your Power and How to Use It" is available from OEP..

we've been trying with him to give him an idea so that; it will be easier for you to work with at home, but if you look at that single arrow in the middle (and I usually draw a square kind of thing around it, to isolate it because otherwise it looks like it might go with the other two arrows to the right of it, that was just our problem in reproducing, this) but that single arrow would be on a 3 x 5 card. This is done not to reproduce what they see but to do something with what they see, to manipulate this short term memory, to do something about it, where the instruction would be, I'm going to show you an arrow. I want you to draw it on your paper as though it were turned a quarter turn to the right." This is the manipulation of immediate visual recall. The child is then started this way and we tell them, "As he shows you he can handle this, you might draw another one at an angle, and then try two." I pointed out yesterday what we have seen not only with children but with adults, when you start having relationships here with two arrows in a very simple arrangement, how an adult even can manipulate this, rotate this but do it in piecemeal form and come up with an entirely different pattern relationship without necessarily recognizing it until they begin to talk about it. So we let the parents realize these things can happen.

One other thing is pointed out, on step 7 there's a suggestion that this could be done with parquetry blocks. This activity is not used --this flash card-- on all of the children that we work with. It depends on what we've seen in terms of their handling the Lyons and Lyons P series, whether or not they've been able to deal with this. If they've dealt with it really effectively, there are other things that I can go to that may be a little bit more useful for the same amount of time put in on it. But where the child has shown us some degrees of—I think of it as visualization in inflexibility, of difficulty in dealing with differences in point of view, difficulties for example even—and you can see it—in a Brock Stereo Motivator or with the quoits Vectogram.

The ring on the basic stereo motivator unit slide 1 can be shifted in space forward or backward of the rabbit and the carrot. We ask them to take a look at this, see it in space with their anaglyphs and to describe it. I'll say, "Well that's easy, the ring is in front and the rabbit and carrot are in the middle on the screen." And then we'll say, "Now describe it as though you were looking at it from the other side." And when we get blanks on this sort of thing, this is the kind of individual that we would probably continue to do things like this with in this way. So that he continues to have opportunities to explore this manipulative aspect of visualization. It's not always enough to get to the point of visual recall and visual memory which, as we normally utilize it, is of short term anyway, and let it go at that. This is one of the reasons why during the training we have them do other things while they are handling short-term visual memory and visual recall. Such as walking; they have to walk to the chalkboard after they've seen the exposure. Such as talking to us while they're walking to the chalkboard about what color it was, because even here we may use anaglyphs even though we're not exposing it in terms of filtering from one system to the other. We're simply having red/green color mixing but we're asking them about what color it was while they're walking to the chalkboard to put it on the chalkboard. We want them to be able to manipulate other systems while they're still dealing with the short-term visual memory. If they can't do this easily and effectively during the training, then we go to this for continuation of this idea.

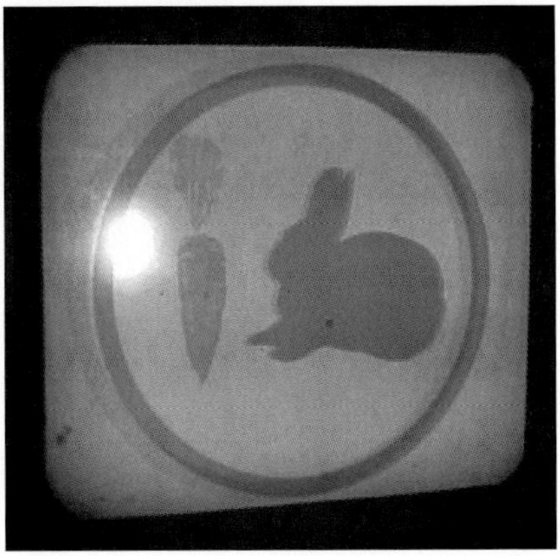

Figure 3: Above is the Brock Stereo Motivator slide number 1. The rabbit and the carrot appear on one slide and are fixed. The top and the bottom of the carrot act as suppression controls. The rings each are on different slides and they can be slid one over another to change the base in and base out demand.

On the tic-tac-toe patterns, we tell the parent, "This is another way we can deal with this sort of visualization or manipulation aspect of visualization. For example, one way you could do it would be to play the tic-tac-toe game back and forth. Let the child start it out. See if he gets the idea that if he puts his "X" in the center that he as often as not has a better chance to win. Don't tell him this." But we tell the parent to avoid putting it in the center themselves. And play the game back. Now the child would expose this to the mother. "Ready now?" he would say, and the mother would put down the "X" on her tic-tac-toe pattern, then she'd put an "O" on hers and flash it back to him, and they'd play this kind of flash tic-tac-toe. We illustrate that with the first tic-tac-toe item as a possibility.

The second one, we say, "Make up a series of cards that would have a winner on them. Flash this card to him but you say to him, I don't want you to put all of the "X's" or "O's" that might be there, down. I simply want you on your tic-tac-toe board to indicate the winning segment, whatever it may be." So this is what he would do after he saw it. We'd tell them, "We also want you to embed some of the pattern. In other words, don't have them all just hanging out where there's nothing to relate it to or see the likes and differences between, but to draw the winning pattern out of other figures. The more you embed it, the harder it becomes when you begin to flash. But all he's to do is to pull out the particular aspect of the total figure that you're looking for. Do something else about it—draw a line in the right direction."

The other thing we do, on the 3rd one in if you'll notice, there is one that's an almost winner. What we do here would be to say to him, "Now you're "O" man this time. I want you to put your "O" in the best possible place, whether it's like so or embedded as "O" man and the parent goes, "Ready, now." What he's to do on his pattern is put the "O" in line with the other "O's". That's all. He's doing something about what he saw rather than duplicating what he saw. Supposing on the same exposure, the same card in the same orientation, the parent now changes the instructions to the child and says, "You're the "X" man. This time, I want you to put an "X" in the best possible place." Now on this flash exposure, the child sees exactly the same pattern, exactly the same spatial relationships, puts a mark in exactly the same place but for an entirely different reason. This is the kind of thinking, processing, manipulative aspect or visualization that we're looking for, that he can deal with some spatial relationships, some information relative to sorting out some likes and differences and now do something with it. Maybe this is belaboring the issue of the thing, but this is the way we do it with the parent to be sure that they understand what it is we're after. That we are not simply after a parroting, reporting of exactly what he has seen. We want him to do something about what he has seen in this flash.

This is the way flash card would be used with those children whom we feel still need more of this kind of activity. The next one is

"Apell Reading." There is a reprint, or there was at least, from the Optometric Weekly some several years ago of two short activities suggested by Dr. Richard Apell [14] and these two activities are abstracted from those two articles. We do much more with the child on the "B", the 2nd one, "Trick Reading." We use "A" also and suggest that when the child is ready, if he is not ready at this point, that the parent then can begin to do this one, too. But we do this "A" part—"Silent-Oral Reading"- to demonstrate to the parent what we're looking for and what is going to be necessary to approach if the child is ever going to get to the point of being able to read and comprehend simultaneously. Because some of these children do read but they do not comprehend. Others can kind of comprehend but they misread and miscall information. They're more global in that sense, and you pin them down to the specifics of the words and they'll read the words much more accurately and not comprehend. This is what we see when we ask them to do these things.

What we need is more flexibility. Let's describe the flexibility that we're talking about. If you will read, I wish we could do it out loud the way I have the parent do, because that's what I have the parent do. I'll do it for you as the parent. I ask the parent to read step (1) under Method under Silent-Oral Reading. I state before they read it that I want them to become aware of the lag between their voice and where their eyes are looking. And then I have them read it. They say, "While reading aloud, become aware of the lag between your voice and where you are looking" Usually by then I can stop them and say, "Did you notice where your eyes were looking while you were talking?" We've reached the end of the line. Usually as I watch their eyes, by the time they are saying "lag" or "between," I see their eyes switch over to the beginning of the next line. Many of the parents are not aware that this is what they're doing in their oral reading, so we'll do it again and this time they begin to be aware of it. I say, "All right, let's try it another way now. This time, I don't want you to move your eyes from the word you're saying until you've said it, but keep going." They start out like this, "While reading aloud, become aware of the lag between --"[15] and by then they usually get the idea. They don't know what they're

---

14. Apell RJ. "Two Techniques Useful in the Training of Retarded. Readers," The Optometric Weekly 56, No. 26 (1965)

15. In this instance Dr. Swartwout would read this in a much choppier and stilted way, as there would be little flow in his reading.

reading, they've read every word very accurately and precisely but they don't know what they're reading. They begin to lose comprehension. I say, "Does it sound familiar?" This is what educators call word calling. This is maybe what we've heard with this particular child that we're working with. He may not quite be ready to take the notions out of this particular thing yet as to how to begin to break into this, but as we move along with him over the next several months, if he does have a sufficient sight vocabulary, he should begin to free up this system, if our visual training in these manipulative aspects of visualization begin to work, where we free up these possibilities. We're dealing with other systems simultaneously and yet with differentials in time and space, because there is a difference between where I'm looking and where I'm saying, and that's spatial. There's a difference also in the timing of the thing, and yet there has to be an integration of the two at the same time. Likes and differences simultaneously. I keep hearing this at seminars and courses that I've gone through at the Gesell Institute. And for a long time I heard it and I didn't quite get the point or didn't quite really comprehend what it was that Dr. John Streff kept trying to press upon us, that we have to deal with these kinds of things. There's a great deal of bipolarity in almost any of these things that we do, like right-left, top-bottom, near-far, central-peripheral, speech-auditory, visual-verbal—all these things that need putting together. And yet there has to be a considerable degree of freedom within and between these systems in order for them to work efficiently. You can see it in terms of comprehension versus word-calling.

So, what we tell the parent is, "This is what we want you to understand about what reading is as we look at it, some of the physiology of it. That your identification focusing is in one place but your speech is in another place and until you can free this up, you have problems in reading. So what we want you to do with him now is "Trick Reading", the one down below, where you will both have the same reading material to work from and you as a parent are going to read this material aloud to the child but you're going to goof it up purposely. You're going to change words, you're going to change "is" to "was", "boy" to "girl", "house" to "home", "Jack" to "Jill"—I mean, don't make it tough on yourself—change the tense of the verb, the action of the verb, the type of adjective, something simple, easy for yourself. Otherwise, you're going to give yourself away if you become too fancy with the thing. What the child is to do is, with the same reading material, be looking and matching what he's hearing and recognize immediately the mismatches between what he's hearing and seeing. This is what we're asking him to do—to recognize a mismatch as immediately as possible between what he's seeing and hearing.

You see, the only thing that's left out of this now is his own speech, his own verbalization of what he is seeing. But we can turn the tables on this one, as we do on many of the activities where we say to the parent, "Now let him assume your role in the activity and let him monitor you, let's reverse the situation. Let's deal with it from the other point of view." I point out further on this particular one, when the child is asked to read in words that are different from the words there, make sure he too knows not to get too fancy with them. Make it easy and simple or he's going to give himself away by hesitation before he says the word. I point out to the parent, too, that in doing this, we're really asking him to do something very difficult and I liken it to the clown on ice who makes it look very easy. But if he weren't very clever and very expert in his work, he could probably break his neck. It's very difficult to be a clown. It's a high skill, and that's what he's asked to do. He's asked to clown a skill, so he has to have some ability to do it. But the very fact that he's thinking about doing it and thinking about creating match versus mismatch, he's dealing with the concept that we want him to work with. This is one of the ones that would be assigned to many of these children who are not secure yet in their reading.

The next one is "Creature Matching." Creature matching is something I ran across through an optometrist in Pennsylvania and found out through him that it was put together by an optometrist in New York State who got it from some educator and then we lost the source, but we still had some of the things in the office so we simply ran them off ourselves. What it amounts to is a series of likes and differences to be recognized simultaneously. On the first sheet, the first line has open symbols; the second line has closed symbols. It says "Creature Matching." There are some 16 pages, I guess in the thing. These are called "Gligs." It says, "All of these are gligs." And then it says in the next line, "None of these are gligs." And then

All of these are Gligs.

None of these is a Glig.

Which of these are Gligs?

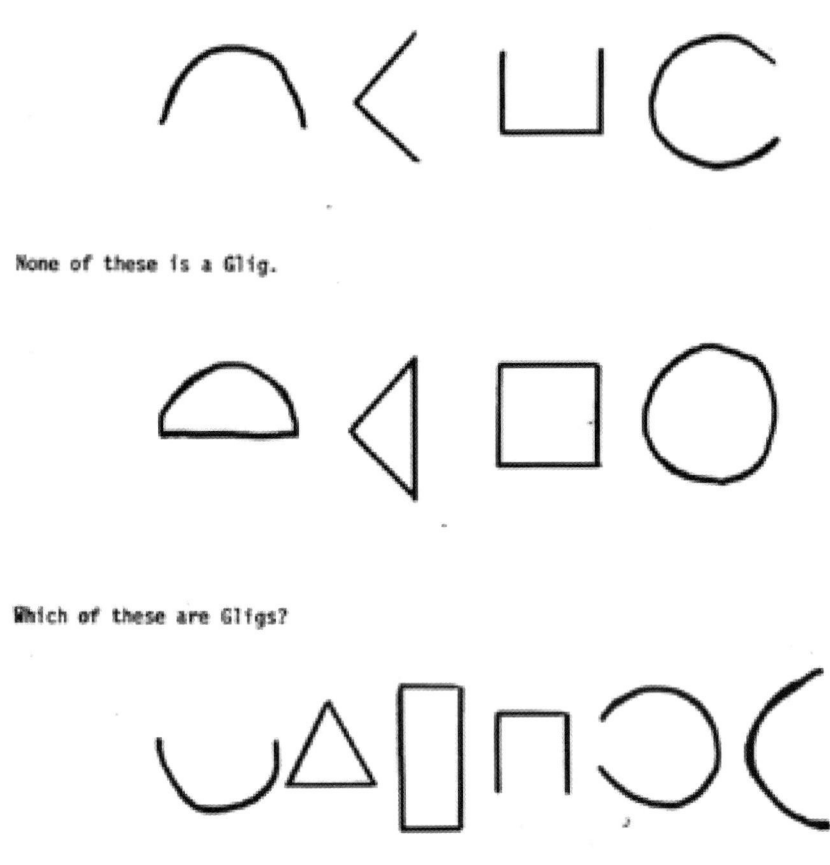

Figure 4: *Gligs as mentioned in the text.*

it says, "Which of these are gligs?" The 3rd line has both open and closed symbols. The child and the parent are asked to pick out those figures in the 3rd line that are gligs. Now if you can see it from back there, you'll see the difference, because there is a great deal of similarity, but there are differences. The differences are open figures versus closed figures. The child would be expected then to point out the open figures on the bottom or 3rd line as the gligs.

We tell them to go through this thing and simply point the things that fit. We give them a workbook. This is one of the statements that would be made at this point. This is going to be reminiscent of some of the activities of the classroom since it's kind of a workbook sort of thing that he will work from, the way they do in school sometimes. And point out to them that it's sort of like school—you're going to play a game with a workbook. This thing goes on and they become more and more complicated, to the point where I have sat down with this, and I remember the first time I saw it, there was one page in there I just couldn't get. I went back to it later on and I managed to get it. I feel confident that there are still some pages in here, that if I went through them right now, I would still have to stop and think and reflect and search out these likes and differences that are simultaneously exposed on the pages. It's a problem-solving task at a high visual level constantly, even when you've gone through it two or three times—not the easier ones, but as you go through it, you'll find that there are then two factors that have to be factored out and three factors that have to be factored out as likes and differences. Some of them will have two on the non-items, will have two perhaps of the three factors and look an awful lot alike, yet there's a small difference. It's these likes and differences, simultaneously exposed to be sorted out and then found among the group that also have now these same likes and differences. As I say, it's hard enough sometimes just to see what the differences are between those two, no less start sorting them out from down below. The kids have a great time with it and so do the parents. These pages are available, but the only place they're available right now as far as I know would be if you wrote to me. We have them copied by a company that puts together all of our material that we work from. Some we mimeograph ourselves but a lot of it we put together this way.

Incidentally, on this we tell them that they don't have to go through the whole thing. Sometimes that's almost a problem because once they get started on it they'd like to go through the whole thing. But each day, in other words, they'd spend maybe up to 10 minutes or do a couple of pages a day. The parent is reminded again at this point, "Remember now, the first day on the 11th week, you're going to do one of these things; the second day you may do this one; the third day you're going to do something else." He's not going to do this every day but he's going to do it, nonetheless, in a continuing way through the next couple of months. About every 3rd to 24th day, he'll get this, about every 3rd to 24th day he gets the other. It's kind of a round-robin through the whole 10-week series.

The next one is "Experience Reader." Now as far as I know, this is strictly from education. I ran across it years ago in a form similar to the way you'll see it here. It had been put out for office use by some other optometrist. I've long since forgotten—most of our material is borrowed from optometrists and I forget quickly from whom, that I can feel more competent that I developed it myself. But I really do forget sometimes. I didn't want to forget Dr. Richard Apell, that's why I called that one "Apell Reading." He's too close to home. I might run into trouble. But "Experience Reader," really, I forget where I got this thing but I do think in the meantime that I've seen it in education. It looks to me more like a kind of thing educators should use. In talking to some of the people I do in education and some of the parents, I find that some of the children have been exposed to this kind of reading in school.

For those who haven't and are not being exposed to it, we will assign it. The kids we work with and the kids who would be having this assigned are children who have a very low ability in sight recognition, being able to identify visually the visual word. Now I say the visual word because they can identify the spoken word of the same meaning. The sound of the symbol, they can identify. They can say it and they use these words in their own vocabulary. A lot of these kids have a very good speech vocabulary and listening vocabulary ability, but they can't read the same words they can understand by ear. They can't read the same words they speak in their daily language. So, this is the idea of this one. Have the child tell them a story when he comes in from school. He can make it up; it can be out of the blue if he wants to. It can be about an experience at school. It can be about a trip they've been on; it can be anything, anything at all, but it should be in their own words. But the parent is advised, as it states in the -write-up about it, not to impose their thinking on him, not to change his sentence structure or his way of use of words, or to correct his English, or in any way alter what he has said. Simply try to write it down just as he has said it.

Now a lot of the parents apparently do type, from my experience with them, and some of them type well enough that they can get it right out on the typewriter. If they can't, I say, "After you've gotten it scribbled down, then write it as best you can so that he can read it. If necessary, print it. Or if you don't type fast but can get it typed, do it immediately—not 10 minutes from now or an hour from now, but immediately—and have him now read it right back." So he reads back the story that he has told. You know, we have gotten the report from one mother just a short while back. This was a 13-year-old youngster, the boy said when he finished reading this thing, within one or two minutes of the time he had said it, "I never said all this." He didn't even recognize the thing, but he read it, and he was reading some words in there that he normally wouldn't identify. The mother, in telling me about this, said, "You know, I really did put it down exactly as he said it, but he didn't make good matching between what he was seeing and what he was hearing after coming through another system." When you see these things and hear these things, no wonder we have problems in getting them to match. If we can start out with an input that we know he can deal with, at least on two other sensory levels because he has produced it in his own speech-auditory monitoring system to come up with the words that are there, that we do find that they begin to make some transfer between the words that they have in their spoken vocabulary and transfer to their reading vocabulary. That, in essence, is the idea, as you'll read in the six statements as to how the parent does it at home.

The next activity sheet on this is "Visual Tracking." This is from the tracking programs at the University of Michigan.[16] I'm sure some of you are familiar with them and some of you may be using them. We've been using them now for about 14 years and within the past year the visual tracking workbook manual has come out in red ink.[17] We now have an additional tool in using it with anaglyphs, especially when we have children who are still showing suppression,

---

16. *These have been also call the Ann Arbor Letter Tracking series and were available with reusable ink systems for a period of time. The easiest way to get these for use with your patients now is to purchase VisionBuilder ™ which is sold by OEP. One of the modules in VB allows you to make new letter tracking activities at random with different size fonts and spacing.*
17. *NOTE: You can print from VisionBuilder ™ in red ink on most laser or inkjet printers as a replacement for this.*

Iln chako evi nomd zeby thipg nare. Zuth pirm nuroc dif stok. Nileg myt lolf. Tixs nom raus zab tuin lugah. Marb seqt rotsir puje. Yonak nesud voz alee. Xart chod bugm turh sref trea gen foru. Vab reps tique kowj. Dagh neulb fwer ilg sida. Ubc they bouf yet neiph vaik. Wolen kig peab nad tenc xerb. Rait rebey fal zibt

Figure 5: Sample letter tracking paragraph with the alphabet hidden in order

who are still showing lack of consistency in circuiting between the two systems, a lack of matching or however you wish to put it. We'll find that there will be differences in timing, differences in ability and speed and consistency in doing these tasks between the two eyes. We may still see it on our tachistoscopic test of digit span at the 10th session that he's still superior in tach response with right eye over left or vice versa. But in this we can continue now systematically throughout the next two or three months a stimulation of information processing through one circuit, the other circuit, and both circuits.

And yet, even when it's only the one on the print, it's pointed out to the parents that he still sees the page with both eyes. He still sees the pencil and his hand that he's using, with both eyes. It's only the central detail, the figure itself, the word, the letters, that he sees with one eye. Both eyes are still working, but one eye is isolated in terms of the centering, and you reverse to the other. I normally write on this particular worksheet that they take home with them, "Spend no more than 10 minutes with this activity." This is reinforcement, I tell them, for the other activities that they're doing. In our noticing of these things in the office, we would have put a little number "11" up on the upper right of all of these. Each week we make assignments for the parents so that they can organize the material through time. The week's visit number is put at the upper right. All of the activities that were assigned on the first week are marked "No. 1." And on my checklist that I keep in the folder, they're also marked and dated so that I also know which ones were assigned the date and which weekly visit. But this one would be marked "11." For all of the ones marked "11," they are reminded, "don't spend more than 10 minutes on these activities. And on this particular one, I want you to use the red/green glasses on two of the units." A unit in this is maybe a paragraph or two of material that looks very much like words, sentences, and yet they're nonsense. They're nonsense words, for those of you who haven't seen it, and I'll leave it up here for any of you who want to look at it later.

The child is asked to go through this and seek out the alphabet in sequence, circling or scratching out or underlining—first the "a" and they move right along and find the first "b", "c", "d" and so on. Now supposing he gets lost in the alphabet. We've assigned this kind of thing on children who haven't been able for three to four years of tutoring to learn the alphabet, and find that within the first month or so that they have learned the alphabet; because there is a built-in monitoring system for them to match against at the top of the page where the alphabet is there in sequence. But they're still having to identify the letters and seek them out and pull them out of ground, but at the same time know the sequence, know what has gone past, which are no longer significant, what is the next significant one. They're dealing with a lot of processing of other things. One little boy took 15 minutes to do the first item. Now we have most of the kids come in and do this in less than two minutes, even as quickly as 50 seconds. This little boy took 15 minutes to seek out the alphabet. This is one of the kids who couldn't even recite the alphabet but who was able to after he had worked on the thing. His time within about a month—good for him—came down to about 5 minutes.

There's one other thing that's built in now that we emphasize very strongly to the parent as being vitally important in this thing, and that is that there is no one line in any of these units without at least one letter in the sequence of finding the alphabet. We want them to be aware of that. Do you see why? We want them to be aware or other information, of other monitoring possibilities of what they're doing. That if they are so highly centered on goal approach that all they're going to do is to find the next letter and the next letter—they can go on two or three or four lines and never realize that they have even—that they're still in a wild-goose chase. They can maintain a broader awareness of the total task, of the process that they're using, of some of the rules and regulations that may be involved in doing what they're doing and not just the goal, that freezes up these thinking aspects of what they're seeing and doing about. So that now we want them aware that if they goof, they have a built-in immediate consequence that they can be aware of for the error in whatever the identification was. I point out to the parent that on the 2nd line there are a "c" and a "d". It's very easy for the child to skip over that "d", having perhaps seen it as a "b" and he'll go on to the next line and there will be no "d" in that line. He shouldn't have to go on three or four lines before he's aware that something is wrong and then have to go all the way back to the beginning, because he's underscored the "c" as the last one. If he goes one line without a "d", he should go right back to the "c" immediately and move on from there to see where it was. He's missed it. He should have this facility of freedom to recognize error in his own processing.

So, this is one that's used. I think I did begin to say about how we used the anaglyphs and didn't complete that. They use the anaglyphs for at least two of these units, with red on right and the other one with red on left. And then they do two more units without the anaglyphs on, just with their own learning lenses—if it doesn't take them more than 2 1/2 minutes to do them. If it takes the child five minutes to do one of the units, then we tell them not to do more than two of them until the time is right. If he can do it later on, next time maybe he can do it in three minutes and then he can do three of them. But don't spend any more than 10 minutes. In other words, do either—spend as much time as 10 minutes on it or do 2 of these units and that's enough for one day.

The last item on these assignments usually would not be sent out at the same time the visual tracking is sent out. I don't do it that way, at least. I mean, I see no reason why someone couldn't do it that way. This, too, is from the Michigan Tracking Program. It's called "Word Tracking." There are a couple of types of things used in this. On the first page, very simply for example, there are five short sentences. One of them says, "The man walked." Underneath it are three lines. The first line says, "she, this, that, them." The second line says, "me, may, mad, man." The 3rd line says, "talked, waked, walked, walled." What he's asked to do, "Read the sentence - **the man walked**- -and now find the words that match the words in the sentence." Out of that first line of "she, this, the, them," he must find the word "**the**" to match the first word in the sentence. But these other words are similar words. These have likes and differences that may be a little bit confusing to this youngster. He is now on an immediate task where he is asked to sort out some of these things. He has an immediate matching monitoring built-in system for it because no one takes away the sentence form. The "the" is there. The "she" is right there, too, but along with the "this" and the "them" is the "the". Can he pull that out to match? Can he see the two that have the immediate and greatest similarity against the others that are a little different? And the same with "man" when he's asked to locate that one out of the other words in that line—"me, may, mad, man".

I frankly went a long time before I even felt the least bit comfortable about using things like this. Because I had to wait until I was sure in my own mind that I could see optometry in what I was doing in this. But likes and differences, identification, and where we've had a child where his focusing mechanism, the accommodation as a piece of physiology has been tight, has been almost inflexible—and so many of these kids are right down, almost to the point of emmetropia, if not emmetropic, where their 19 (accommodation tested in the phoropter monocularly and binocularly) findings do show very poor flexibility, as do any of the other findings that we're looking at with accommodation involved. This is a physiological movement system, and any movement system that becomes tight and stressed, as far as I'm concerned, is not going to be that effective in its operation, in the purposefulness, in the activities that it's to be used for. We do say that one of the major functions of accommodation is to control the system which we also refer to as identification, information processing. If it lacks the freedom for movement, is tight and stressed, I don't think I have the kind of physiology going for me to utilize on the kind of discrete manipulations that are going to be necessary in reading, and combining that part of physiology with the transportation system, the skeletal movement, the saccades, the pursuits and all the other things that are necessary. Because that accommodation system as physiology is utilized for identification, not just of the words that this kid's looking at. How you know this and I know this but I can forget it sometimes and I no longer do. That while he's reading these words, whatever they are—this is the word, let's say, that identification-wise he's reading. You know what else he's doing at that time, too. He's also processing localization information as we were talking about it the other day so that he can get to the right place at the right time while he's still dealing with words. We were talking about how we have to free up these systems in order to still do this and have comprehension. The guy who can't do this is the one who keeps losing his place. He misses his words, he skips over things, he's having difficulty in moving these movement aspects of the system for identification and localization simultaneously in order to process the information and be at the right place at the right time predictively. It has to all happen at once.

We also say that under stresses—and I'm talking about stresses in the accommodative physiology—that it's tightened up. That if this physiology tightens up, or this physiology tightens up, my perceptual fields are going to constrict—period. I'm not going to be in a good position to sit down and read. I'm not going to be in a good situation to sit down and communicate even. This then is important for me, because I see the physiology in this kind of likes and differences, matching simultaneously as well as the differences between words. He may have to do this, and he may only be able to do this if he has his training lenses on. Or his learning lenses that he's using in school. This is emphasized to the parent, that he's not to do this without them, because most of these children by the time they've reached this stage, they're getting more benefit from those lenses that they've had prescribed perhaps before the program started. We now want to use these lenses to protect these more fragile skills that are beginning to develop in these movement patterns that we're beginning to measure in the accommodative physiology that is being used for information processing, both space localization and symbol identification. These things have to go on simultaneously and I don't want to put him on more of this kind of stuff without that lens protection. This is, as I see it, our role in doing a thing like this.

This then, they do a page or two of this on maybe the 4th day or the 5th day. This is often assigned when they come back for the progress evaluation, if they have done well with the visual tracking; that is, seeking out the alphabet. I'll leave that up here, too, for anybody who wants to see it. Those are, for the most part, the special items.

MEMBER: I'm a teacher. I've observed that I sometimes have trouble with the child who has reading lenses or learning lenses to keep them on or to remember to put them on during certain reading near point tasks, and my observation has been that the child with the bifocal design is much less a problem this way and generally tends to have them on at the right time in the classroom.

DR. SWARTWOUT: This was my observation, too, and that goes back almost 20 years of the 21 I've been in practice. We tried it also with single vision lenses at that time and ran into the same problem on our progress examinations, that they weren't being used appropriately, they were being forgotten much of the time, they would be taken off to see the chalkboard and be forgotten to be put on again, because so much of it is near-far looking anyway. It's just a customary way of handling things in most of our offices today; I would presume that we're using bifocal lenses. But apparently you're still seeing some with single vision reading lenses. It's not doing a favor to the child and it's not doing a favor to the teacher who's trying to go along with this concept of supporting these skill areas under this kind of contained, sustained, intense work. It's much easier for the child. It's harder for the parents to accept, sometimes, but it's easier for the child to accept in the bifocal form.

I frequently, going through some of these things that we use and activities in the office, emphasize the concepts more than the actual technique, utilizing some procedures as illustrations of how we use technique. But more to the point of some of the concepts that we've tried to incorporate with our optometric procedures, so that we're working from a broader base. I sometimes find myself being misunderstood. That perhaps we don't really use lenses very much, that these things are all being done without lenses. I wouldn't want that kind of impression to be heard, and since it has been brought to my attention at least twice within the past few hours, that one of the comments was rather late and one rather early, about our use of lenses in training. I think most of you do have an idea that I do use lenses. I use them in testing, I use them in training, I use them for prescription, I use them for control, and I use them to disembed. I use them to stabilize and I use them to rearrange conditions so that I can begin to get at something.

One of the things that I've alluded to here, and I did it this way specifically to point out how we use a lens to help develop some additional ranges and flexibilities in this accommodative physiology, and at the same time as these things develop, to begin to spread or to control rather some of the skills that begin to develop out of this. The ability of a child to do this sort of thing I'm describing here, being able to read words and localize at the same time, is a demonstration that you can frequently utilize with your young adults, teenagers, even some of the more sharp young children, where you can ask them to look back and forth from the end of the line to the beginning of a line with and without the lenses you're going to prescribe. They can communicate to you, yes, they see a difference, that they've slowed down without the lenses on. They're not able to move their eyes as efficiently, as smoothly, as accurately or rapidly without the lens that you're prescribing at near. It's pointed out to the parents at this point that although, generally speaking, most people think of lenses in terms of clarity and producing sharper identification of words, letters and symbols, that here we're seeing a result of a lens upon the movement of the eyes. I point out that the reason for this is that he's taking a bigger bite of information. And if you don't believe this, try this with the MacDonald Form Field Letter chart[18] on this child who is able to look back and forth faster. Because many times this is so obvious that you can see the movement as you watch the eyes. When you move the lenses away, you'll see the undershooting, you'll see the slow-down. Let him look at the little "V" in the center of the MacDonald Form Field chart and ask him about the rest of the field, the letters, while he's looking through the lens. Then remove the lenses and watch the wow kind of expression. It doesn't happen all the time but it happens enough of the time that we use it quite a bit in the office, and with adults, too. In pre-presbyope, for example, where they're working hard, yet they really aren't there for a complaint, they're there because they're good patients and they schedule this periodic re-examination anyway. And here you can do something in the near area and show them why we want to do it, that they're going to be able to deal with a bigger bite of information and at the same time get more information in space at the same time and to be more predictive of the movement patterns and still identify what they're looking at. So, it eases off the stresses of the system.

We use lenses like this to protect and control this very delicate physiology of accommodation while we're going through the training, because we're going to be putting it under some additional stresses in order to get movement, in order to get some of the direction in

---

18. *This was a chart done by the late Dr. Lawrence MacDonald. This can be purchased from OEP as MacDonald Form Recognition Field Cards (100 pack).*

change that we're looking for. We would also do this to increase awareness. We are using lenses to increase awareness and sensitivity to spatial shifts and spatial relationships. We do things like this, matching it with hand, for example in accommodative rock, when we're discussing SILO, where the individual may be under dissociation with plus and minus. We usually do this standing, incidentally. We use a light box on our reading bar, on our reading stand. They stand with a phorometer here, with the lenses and dissociation, the target out there and they describe it. Many times we'll find that we can help them recognize some of the mismatches within their identification systems.

For example, when they look at the upper target and they say, "That one is small and closer and the bottom one is big and far away," and they're reaching like this. Then we ask them, "This in smaller and closer and you're reaching out here?" Somehow, visually, they're seeing this spatial projection differently than they feel it. We'll get mismatches like this between where they are reaching and where they say they're seeing. If they can begin to feel these things themselves, they can begin to look at some of their own monitoring systems.

This is the same kind of thing I mentioned yesterday, that we also use a metronome with, incidentally, to help with the rocking aspect of accommodation. Different things will begin to help in the identification, but we certainly have to use lenses in this way of developing this awareness of spatial shift and relationships. We also want to use lenses to develop greater range and freedom between the accommodation and the convergence systems. This is part of what we are talking about here. This can best be done, I think, if we can relate it with identification and localization. How best can we get at this than though the use of lenses, minus or plus, and prisms also. One of the other things that we use lenses for in the training is to develop awareness of the internal postural and gravitational aspects of the organism. Have you tried, for example, on a very tight kid where you're getting very little movement and you can't get them freed up particularly in his/shoulder even, the neck, the head, all these areas real tight, put low power plus/minus; like a -0.50 on the right and a +0.50 on the left and watch them begin to rotate, and switch them around and watch them begin to rotate. The body will move on the basis of alteration of input at the visual level in this kind of asymmetry to get some movement. We will do this while they're reading sometimes, binocularly, in other words, without rocking. It's a binocular exposure but flip a -0.50 and a +0.50 around, or -0.25 and a +0.25 around from one eye to the other so that they are getting kind of a spatial rock, but you'll see the effect in terms of movement patterns of the body.

The same thing is true with prisms. We use prisms more and more we find in our training. Much of it is bilateral based, That is, bilaterally base-up or bilaterally base-down[19], bilaterally to the right or left, while they're doing other things, to create purposely in this way a mismatch between the visual, postural, gravitational, hand, projection systems. Just as we do in a Cheiroscope, we do this and don't think anything much about it, that we're creating mismatches here. But these are purposely created mismatched systems so that the individual can explore some of the possibilities within this system for identification and matching up other systems. We can do it right out in the room with other activities, with lenses and prisms. We use this. All the activities that we use in the office, on each of the activity sheets for each week, there is a space for me to indicate for each particular patient what particular lenses I want the assistant to use that particular day on that particular activity. We do not use a one specific training lens power like let's say +1.00 or +1.50 or +0.50 as a specific training lens for a specific case. We use a range, generally, and I would indicate on the worksheet that the assistants work from what this individual's working training lens ranges are going to be. For example it might be +1.25, + or -0.50. There may be something very specific. When dealing with distance activities, +2.00. I may want to blur this fellow because he is full of hot spots out here, so we would lose the organization of the periphery so he could begin to concentrate a little bit better on a central area. Or we might do certain activities with the wall-climbing child; the one all over the place. We might put excessive minus on this child for certain activities, to help to move him in to center, but this is a movement into center in a different way, for a different purpose. We would use a different kind of lens. This couldn't possibly be utilized as a prescription lens, even though we could see it, perhaps, slowing

---

19. *The more conventional term for this use of prisms now is "yoked"; both prisms pointing in the same direction.*

down, pulling it on center. He may even be able to walk and stand on a balance board this way, or walking rail, or things of this sort.

But we think more in terms of developing flexibilities in the use of the training lenses because I'm still thinking in terms of the flexibility I want in this physiology; that I want him to be able to deal with information processing of all kinds under many different kinds of conditions. Because he's not going to have a block box of silence with only a lighted environment to deal with that's of a particularly easy nature in any of his school work or any of his homework. We also use contact lenses in our visual training. I saw some fascinating visual training cases that couldn't have turned out the way they did unless we had the availability of contact lenses to work with. I'm thinking of some of the myopia cases. I'm thinking particularly of some of the anisometropia cases and also of post trauma rehabilitation where we've been able to work some very interesting results, but only because we had the availability of contact lenses. Lenses are an intimate and integral part of it. They're the basis of anything that I do in visual training. I work from there as a base and I kind of leave it out of the general discussion because I figure that's the real optometry. What I've been talking about is how we can elaborate our real optometry from an analytical understanding of the effect of a lens upon this particular organism, and move it into some other concepts that are available to us from other disciplines, like education, psychology, learning theory, pediatrics, and what-have-you. These people also are doing some things that are right, just as we are doing some things that are right. There are a lot of us who are doing things right, but in different regards. The broader we can make our base, the broader we can help the child develop his base and the faster and more effectively we're able to carry out our programs.

By involving it, not just in the office but at home, by beginning communication with the schools; and there are ways to do that. I would recommend one, aside from usual reporting, especially where the teacher, as I find in the last year or so, requests through the parents oftentimes, "Is there any information that the doctor can give me that I may use in my classroom?" I've really been amazed at this kind of thing. Sometimes it's not a verbal request but a letter to me, handed to the parent to be given to me. What we do is utilize some of the information that is in this past series of chapters by Dr. Hal

Wiener,[20] who gave a very interesting rundown of possible recommendations for some of these children in the classroom. Because here's another report; we surely don't need another report to write out. But if we have a list where we can say to the typist, "1,2,3,4," and she knows now from her list that she keeps by the typewriter that this is the report she's going to get because you've pulled out these particular items for this particular child for the teacher, then this can be a major time saver. We still can pass this information on without it taking another hour or two hours of time on our part.

---

20. Wiener H. *"Vision in the Classroom" OEP Curriculum II Series, 1970-71*

Dr. Paul Dunn (Pediatrician)
The "Team Approach"
Care of Child Vision Problems
1971

I really feel much honored to be speaking at this conference. This is the 35th Annual Conference. Getting down to today's subject, who is this optometric patient that we're talking about? Well first, of course there'd be the adult optometric patient who goes is in his 40's and has various visual problems which optometrists look into and design glasses specifically for him and for his occupation. If he's looking up while doing his work, then he would need a little different type of a lens than the one who is looking straight ahead or looking down in his occupation. But the one that we're primarily concerned with is the pediatric optometric patient. Who is he? He's the child with the neurologically based learning disability. He's the child who cannot feed and develop his intelligence by the usual method, who is unable to process information offered to him by the school. He's the hyperactive uncoordinated child whose eye may be slightly crossed, or holds his place with his finger while he's reading. He's the preschooler who can't stay within the lines while coloring. Or he's the youngster who can't learn to button his own clothes. He may be bright but seems to be unable to concentrate on a near-point task for long periods. He is the child who finally accepts and carries within himself the conviction that he is a clumsy, stupid, nervous problem child. He is the headache and the heartache of every school system in the country. And his kind of problem can be found in 10 to 40% of the current school age population.

So you see, the incidence of the problems that you see in your optometric offices is tremendous. There are a few learning disability statistics that have been compiled that indicate that 25% of 8th grade graduates are non-readers when they graduate. Not just poor readers, but they cannot read. One-third of all high school freshmen drop out before they graduate, and most of these problems are also associated with a very significant functional-visual problem.

What about the pediatrician's viewpoint of these problems? Well, the very common and probably the most current viewpoint of most pediatricians is one that I had when I was in pediatric practice before getting involved in this aspect of pediatrics. When I would see a child do a school exam—we'd use the old Snellen chart, the old 20/20 chart—and we found a child who needed some further consultation, I used to make a special point of saying, "Now don't go to an optometrist. Be sure you go to an ophthalmologist." Nobody ever taught us that, it's just one of those things that you pick up along the way. And of course, since then I've realized how very wrong I was. The future viewpoint of the pediatrician is what we are primarily concerned with and there is a great need for education of students of medicine and optometry and education and psychology and in all the related disciplines—we have to start with educating them so that the viewpoint of future pediatricians is one of communication and understanding of one another's problems and one another's work.

What about the needs of this optometric patient? Obviously, of course, he needs treatment for his problem but maybe even more important than this specific treatment is this communication and cooperation between disciplines in the child professions. The knowledge of how to prevent and correct many of the physical causes of reading and learning difficulties already exist in the various specialty disciplines of medicine, optometry, psychology, education and nutrition—all of the related disciplines already have the knowledge, current technology. The knowledge is already there to solve these problems. It's just a matter of fully integrating and applying the knowledge that already exists. This is absolutely essential if the treatment that the child gets, and the evaluation procedures that he has are coordinated and complete. The treatment should be one which allows his problem to be solved. Not just to help him cope with his problem but to help him get rid of the problem.

Through the years, starting with Itard and Seguin back in the early 1800's, there are real giants in this field. Like the two French physicians, Montessori, Skeffington, Getman, Pay, Harmon, Doman and Delacato, and many others who have contributed. There's also a physical educator in Germany, Dr. Diem, who has made tremendous contributions. If we can coordinate all this, then we are well on the way to solving these problems.

I'd like to spend a little bit of time acquainting you with how I got involved in this. Obviously, with the 10 children we have, you are thrust right into pediatrics right off the bat. I was in graduate pediatric practice but hated to see these kids come in—the child with the learning problem, the child with the more severe brain injury, the so-called cerebral palsy child. We hated to see them come in because we didn't know what to do with them. It wasn't really until about 12 or so years ago (1959) that Mrs. Dunn and I became aware of the Montessori approach to education. We read all we could about it and it seemed like something that should be. We talked with some other physician friends of ours and various others. Then, we started the Montessori school which is now in its 11th year of operation. The same group founded the Illinois Montessori Society. For those of you who may not be familiar, Dr. Montessori was a physician also, whose first work was not really that of a physician but that of an educator. She was assigned to teach a group of mentally defective children in one of the institutions of Rome at that time. She went back to Seguin's work and elaborated on it. After a period of time, she brought these children to a point where they were passing the examinations of the normal public school children. Probably the reason she had such success was that these children were probably brain injured, not genetically defective, but suffering from a brain injury. She was providing them with what we now term neurological organization. She was providing them with a lot of gross motor activity, with a lot of freedom to move, a lot of stimulation of all of the senses and she was following a developmental procedure, much as those of you in developmental optometry are doing.

Behind all of this Montessori activity was a girl who was the sparkplug of the revival of Montessori, Nancy Rambusch. Maybe some of you have met her, a very dynamic, outgoing, articulate woman who came into town one weekend to help us get started. She cornered me on the porch and went on about Doman and Delacato and the work they were doing in Philadelphia and how it all ties in with Montessori. And she just went on and on about normal development and "you've got to find out what they're doing." At a Montessori meeting in Connecticut a while back, Delacato was one of the speakers. We arranged to stop by in Philadelphia on the way back for a short time, and instead stayed two full days and our lives haven't been the same since. You can't be exposed to what they're doing with an open mind and ever again think the same about children, whether they're children with problems or a normal child, or an adult, for that matter, because the concepts apply to man, period, not just to a brain-injured child.

Sometime later, a neurologist friend of ours and I went back and spent some time. During this time, we had seen and heard enough that we felt an obligation to see what happened to children under this program. So we came back and started the Chicago Center for Achievement of Human Potential, working with the children with the more severe problems as well as the child with the learning disability, and now in pediatrics applying these same principles to normal development in what we have instructed mothers to do with their normal babies.

Shortly after World War II, Doman and Delacato and the staff there that consisted of Dr. Temple Fay Dr. Robert Doman, Glen Doman the physical therapist and Delacato who is an educator and psychologist were working with the children with brain injuries. They were using the classical treatment of braces and physical therapy once a week and occupational therapy. But they really weren't getting any place with it. They had very minimal results. In analyzing the situation, they decided that they weren't working hard enough, so they decided to take no more new patients and really go all out in their efforts—physical therapy, 3 or 4 times a day instead of once a week. They tallied up the results and found about 1/3rd of the kids had advanced again a little bit, another 1/3rd stayed the same, and the other 1/3rd had actually regressed with all of this intensive care. This was right in line with the reports of others in the field, like Dr. Zuc and Dr. Johnson. They really made the first report in history of the results of any form of treatment, in which they said that children without any treatment are as likely to do as well as children on this treatment which isn't saying very much. And then three years later, in 1958, Dr. Ingraham reported and their data compared with Zuc and Johnson with the same conclusion. Then Doman and Delacato, in 1960, reported on their results for this treatment compared to their own classical results in the same group of children. In 1962, Richmond Payne, a pediatric neurologist from Harvard reported on their results, and in his report makes the same statement, that children without any treatment at all are as likely to do as well.

You may be wondering why I'm saying so much about the child with the more severe problem. These are not the children that you usually see. But you will understand what we'll be saying about your patients if we spend a little time first on these patients who really exhibit development in very slow motion, and have taught us tremendous amounts; brought us a lot of information that's helpful for these other children. This is very discouraging, of course, to them and even more so when they look at a group of other patients who had been on treatment but for some reason or other, the treatment was stopped. In this group, there were a significant number who had advanced further than the best of theirs had without any treatment at all and none had regressed. So either we find a better way or go into some other business. They weren't about to do this, so they said, "Let's see what we're doing. Why do some of them get worse? Well, here's the problem in the brain, causes the spastic muscles. If we can get that out flat with a brace, we can do something with it, they can at least ambulate." But that doesn't change the spasticity. Now you're applying continuous resistance against the muscle that's already tight, and of course there's a very good possibility that you'll make it tighter and it will come down faster and further than it did before.

So they knew the first thing they were going to do was get all of these appliances out of the way. Since they were interested, mainly, in mobility in the group of 76 children that finally evolved out of it, they said, "Now let's see what happens to these children just by giving them the opportunity to move. Just by putting them on the floor during the waking hours and see what happens." They did this and it wasn't long until things did happen. These children did begin to move out in a way that they hadn't done before. They went so far and they stopped. They stopped in 4 groups. There were those who still had no mobility; there were those who were crawling in a prone position; there were those who were creeping up on their hands and knees; and a few who were walking. And there was no more progress. Then they realized that these were subdivided into those children who were going along without any particular pattern. They would be just moving this arm and that arm and this leg and both legs but they were getting some place. There were those who were going along homologously, that is, both hands coming out this way. There was the homolateral group, that is, the same side, this arm and leg. And then there was the cross-pattern, like we all walk, opposite hand and foot.

It was only at this point that they realized that normal children, if they're given the opportunity to, will go through these same stages in the development of their mobility that was being exhibited by these brain-injured children. Checking the work by Gesell[1] and making various observations on their own for a long period of time, they realized this, which really they had known before if they had just stopped to think about it. So, they reasoned, if normal children do this, maybe it's essential that they go through these progressive stages in development. For development of optimum ability these are related to other aspects of development—to language and division and manual development. So, since these children can't, because of their brain injury and also probably in many cases superimposed sensory deprivation, then let's do it for them. So they began to move the arms and legs in a way simulating what the child would do for himself if he were able, not just as exercise but doing this as another way of programming the nervous system; of putting in these basic inputs, these basic stimuli that the normal baby gets himself from moving about the environment. So it's programming the nervous system, not just exercise, and hoping to get them from one level of development to the other. Not only helping his mobility but, as you know from the four circles in developmental vision, that vision and understanding and language and everything are all tied in with anti-gravity processes or locomotion.

The results of all this, in addition to the patterning, which is this movement of the arms and legs, they also had the children perform these activities in any way that they could. Again this was done not as exercise but as input. Also, they provided opportunity for hearing a lot of speech, for chewing, for blowing, sucking, exercising the tongue, all enhancing the movement of speech. They did functional tests to determine the level of manual development. If they had a prehensile grasp, that level was reinforced and attempts made in many

---

1. *Editor's Note: Arnold Gesell, MD was a pediatrician who worked closely with optometry and authored the book, Vision Its Development in Infant and Child, available from OEP.*

ways to work on the next higher level. The same thing was done in vision, hearing and touch on the input side, reinforcing attained level and working on the next level in a whole variety of ways. The idea is to greatly increase the frequency and the intensity and the duration of sensory input. Hopefully in this way, they will get the reaction within the little black box of the computer and get increased amount of efficiency of motor output in mobility, language, manual competence, with the resultant feedback. Hopefully that will keep this cybernetic loop going, with the ultimate objective of restoring neurological organization and bringing the patient back to as normal a state as possible.

The results in mobility were very significant. They were like this compared to the other results they had with the classical treatment. For example, out of the 76, there were 21 initially who had no mobility at all. Out of these 21, there were 3 at the end of the 2 years who had begun to walk and others who had moved up to crawling or creeping. Still others who started at a higher level moved up to higher levels. So the results were very significant, not only in mobility but also in other areas in which they were working.

What is the relationship of this to the child with the learning disability? The child with the learning problem, even though he grossly looks normal and acts normal, is really, as are all of us actually, on the same continuum. We're all some place on a continuum from deaf at the bottom up through the profoundly brain-injured child to severely, the moderately, the mildly brain-injured, the hyperactive child with a reading problem, the average child, the superior child, and at the top this ideal person; this perfect physical specimen with tremendous mentality and wonderful personality that relates well to everybody. There are some of those people. I was talking about this one time at a talk when Mrs. Dunn was present, and knowing what the reaction would be, I said in talking about this ideal, "You know there are not many of us left anymore." It got the expected reaction, of course.

These children are on the same continuum and we all are some place in there. We all eventually go up and we come back down, so that the basic principles are the same no matter where we find ourselves. What is the rationale of the treatment that we use? One statement is that children who are neurologically well-organized teach themselves. They can teach themselves to a very high level of development. The Quiz Kid, we might say, "Who taught him?" Well, probably nobody taught him, he probably taught a lot to himself. This brings up the story of this boy who was a Quiz Kid, just a little 14-year-old, who really knew a lot about many things. His mother was gone one day, his grandmother was watching over him and he was busy and all of a sudden he said, out of a clear sky, "Grandmother, where did I come from?" She was sort of taken aback and finally recovered and said, "When you were a little baby, a stork flew over your Mother's and Daddy's house and dropped you down the chimney." "Is that right? Do you mean that's really where I came from?" "Yes, that's it." So he seemed satisfied and she was relieved until he said, "Well now, where did Mommy, and Daddy come from?" She wanted to be consistent, so she said, "When they were little babies, two storks flew over and dropped them down their mother's and daddy's chimneys." "You don't mean it! Is that true?" "Yes, that's the way it was." So of course the next thing, "Where did their mothers and daddies come from?" And of course, four storks flew over and dropped them down their mother's and daddies' chimneys. "You really mean it." "Yes Johnny, that's it." So he went over to his desk and got his diary out and wrote feverishly for a minute or so. He closed the book and said, "Grandma, I'm going out to play." She couldn't wait for him to slam the door to find out what he had written. On that day he wrote, "Today, I have made a truly astounding discovery of a very unique physiological phenomena. There hasn't been a normal birth in our family for three generations." So, he was probably well organized neurologically and came up with a lot of information that Grandma didn't know about.

Further on this rationale: The child whose lower mobility patterns (crawling on his stomach, creeping up on hands and knees) are uncoordinated indicates faulty automatic brain mechanisms in lower level neuromotor systems which may interfere with the integrity of higher-level cortical functions of more complex motor tasks or in reading, writing, spelling or thinking. This lack of organization prevents him from automatically transferring input information from his senses into efficient motor output, for example, in hitting an oncoming ball or writing words which are spoken to him or copying simple geometric forms which are shown to him. The cause of such a child's functional disorders in the classroom and on the playground is a neurological dysfunction often associated with an overall maturational lag which becomes apparent very early in his development. If any treatment program is to be fully effective for him, it must be directed toward organizing neural pathways in lower brain levels so that he can integrate incoming sense data with well-established motor patterns efficiently and automatically, and be able to function with optimal efficiency at the higher cortical levels called for in most classroom activities.

Tutoring and special methods are important in getting around the symptoms of a specific learning disability and teaching a child to cope with his limitations once the problem begins to manifest itself during the school years. But only a neurologically organizing motor program will reduce the occurrence of such developmental problems in young children and allow school-age children to rid themselves of their dysfunctions. For the child's nervous system to be well organized and able to help him relate accurately to his environment, he must have adequate opportunity to program his nervous system with basic input from movement and other available sensory experiences. Neural pathways are organized in an orderly progression in a well developing child from a purely reflex level in the newborn up through more complicated levels of integration as a result of the various developmental stages in mobility, language, manual competence as well as visual, auditory and tactile competence.

Basic early inputs may be insufficient or missing completely from the lower levels of the ongoing spiral of development due to a lack of sufficient environmental opportunity or because of an inherited developmental system or developmental pattern that just doesn't allow him to spend sufficient time in some of these early stages of development. Or perhaps due to a brain injury or to some combination, or maybe also have some related nutritional deficit involved in it. Gaps in early functional mobility and motor development thus may manifest themselves again and again as the child's perceptual and then cognitive processes become his more predominant mode of interacting with his environment.

Before going into some of the details of this treatment, I think it might be good to spend a little time with normal development, just like in medical school; the same may be true in optometry school, before a student knows what he's seeing or hearing as abnormal, he first has to know a lot about the normal. Much of what we will be saying, I'm sure, is a little repetitious for you in this audience, but I think it may be in a little different light. There's a very interesting comparison between the development of every human being and the evolution of the whole phylogenetic scale; ontogeny recapitulates phylogeny. Development really reproduces evolution. I could spend a lot of time talking about evolution, too, but recent discoveries, at least in the last 20 or 30 years, show that this did happen.

One very basic, simple statement is that learning is a function of the central nervous system. I hardly need to make that statement. The central nervous system develops in a phylogenetic way. If we go back down the phylogenetic scale to the very simple animal, the fish, we find an animal with a very simple nervous system equivalent to our spinal cord and the medulla in which are located the centers that are essential to life. At birth, a baby has his whole brain but it really isn't functioning for him. Myelin, which you're familiar with, like the insulation around a wire is present only as far as the medulla. There's a little bit that goes up further but for all practical purposes, a newborn baby is a reflex animal. He's a brainstem animal, a brainstem person. His actions are reflex.

Now as you go back phylogenetically again and come up the scale, you get into the amphibians and the reptiles and also a more complicated type of a nervous system equivalent to our heart. What are these animals doing? They're now sprouting extremities, crawling so to speak on their stomach. As myelin is laid down in this direction and the baby now becomes functional at this level, he begins to crawl on his stomach. No pattern, homologously, homolaterally and finally the cross pattern. And now you get up to the quadrupeds. What is this baby doing? Like this animal, he's sort of up on his hands and knees, creeping. Now we get up to the primates, the apes and all of that group, and they're now upright, walking homolaterally, developing prehension and also developing a much greater cortex. Now these animals have a cortex, too, but it's a very inactive one. They're mainly brainstem animals. But now the primates are developing much more. Their eyes are coming around to the front; they're developing manual activities, so to speak. Finally, we come up now to man at the highest level with a much more highly developed cortex and having abilities peculiar to man. Walking in cross pattern, a written meaningful language, the ability to close his thumbs and fingers—initially, do it mentally one side and the other side, then together, then a bimanual function and finally, writing, at the highest level of manual development. We also have then, superimposed on all of this something else that is peculiar to man and that is cerebral dominance. One side or the other of the brain does become the dominant side. If this is the right side and the left side of the brain, you have a right-handed person. The left side is the dominant side because of the crossing over here. You're all familiar with that aspect of it.

Now all of this, the whole central nervous system—the brain, the spinal cord and the peripheral nerves, the input fibers, the output fibers, the end organs—all developed through use. Without use, of course, it doesn't develop. You could have a baby with all the potentials of all the great minds that ever lived but if he didn't have opportunity to move and to have his senses stimulated, he would never develop. He'd be retarded severely and irrevocably if it went on long enough simply from sensory deprivation and lack of the opportunity to move. If he weren't exposed to light, as you well know, he'd be blind, too. The end organs, the muscles, everything; every part of the body develops through use. So, what does this all boil down to? Everything really that we're talking about is based on cybernetics; information, utilization in the solution of the problem that has come in with the whole computer age. That's a very interesting diagram that we can put down here that illustrates some of the terms that you hear in talking with people working with computers. "Garbage in, garbage out," for example. "The little black box"; the brain, the works of the system. Of course, before you get anything out, you first have to program it with input, with energy. What is this mainly in us? Visual, auditory and tactile input. Also the input—we could put "K" here, too—kinesthetic, the input from movement and from our position in space.

Now as these inputs go in, a variety of things happen. They are first stored and then the baby in his development begins to compare one to the other. Then as he notices similarities, he classifies information, all of which is following one or more laws. Now he gets into problem-solving situations and what happens? Well, he recalls previous information that's been stored. If it's a simple problem, he makes a simple judgment on the basis of that and he solves the problem. If it's a more complicated problem to solve, requiring more storage up here, more concepts, more information, more options to use then he has to use strategies. Of course, this results in output or behavior. This goes about the same as mobility, language and manual competence; the way in which we do everything. As a result of that, you get feedback, which in turn affects the input and there is evidence to show that it affects the little black box; within which physical and chemical changes are brought about. I think you can see the relationship of this external cybernetic loop and also the billions of internal loops which are going on within the black box. You can see the relationship of that to the four circles of developmental vision.

Now there's a correction of Rosenzwieg.[2] Their group has done some work which goes back a few years, in which they had two groups of rats, same genetic background so they would have the same potential. The idea was to stimulate one group and see if they learned better than the isolated control. This did happen. The exercised, stimulated group did learn better and also they found that chemical changes took place. There were enzymes activated in the brain of the stimulated animals that were not in the control group. On sacrificing the animals, they found that the brain was bigger; the cortex was thicker by 1 to 2 mm than the isolated control. There were definite physical changes as well as the chemical changes as well as the increased ability to learn, to recall previously learned information, and to learn new information. There's another man who sort of repeated this, but he went one step further—Dr. Altman at MIT.[3] He found the same things but what he did was to inject a radioactive material which was selectively picked up by glial cells in the brain and deposited as a pigmented area in the plasm of the

---

2. *From Wikipedia: Mark Richard Rosenzweig (September 12, 1922 – July 20, 2009) was an American research psychologist who found in animal studies on neuroplasticity that the brain continues developing anatomically, reshaping and repairing itself into adulthood based on life experiences, overturning the conventional wisdom that the brain reached full maturity in childhood.*
3. *From Wikipedia: Joseph Altman discovered adult neurogenesis, the creation of new neurons in the adult brain, in the 1960. As an independent investigator at MIT, his results were largely ignored. In the late 1990s, the fact that the brain can create new neurons even into adulthood was rediscovered, leading it to be one of the hottest fields in neuroscience.*

cell. He found on autopsy of the animals that these glial cells multiplied. The longer the animal had been stimulated, the more glial cells he found and he knew that they were multiplying because they also had the pigmented area. Now the glial cells, you will recall, lie in among the neurons and they've always been known to be important in the nutrition of the neuron and therefore of course in the function of the animal. As these became greater in number, it was often postulated that probably the reason these animals learned better was that the increased glial cells sort of potentiated the transmission of the nerve impulse and therefore made the animal more efficient.

He found something else that was even more startling and that is in relationship to the neurons themselves. We always believed firmly without any doubt, dogmatically believed, that an infant is born with the total number of neurons that he will have the rest of his life, so he'd better make the most of it. But Altman found that this isn't true. He found that 80 to 90% of the micro-neurons that had to do with the thinking process developed after birth and developed in infancy, mainly, and in proportion to the amount of sensory stimulation that the baby receives in his infancy. Now if this is true, we can't afford to ignore it. Not only for the children with problems but also in what we do with our children in their normal cult. The question comes up, well, O.K., so it's true in rats, that doesn't mean that it's true in man. Which is true? It doesn't prove that it's true in man.

Dr. Kresch, I had the opportunity to meet him a few years ago, and he was talking about this as well as some other aspects of it. When this question was put to him, he said, I'll agree, this doesn't prove it's true in man but it's reasonable to assume that it's true in man! I think it would be socially criminal to assume that it is not true in man, and in so assuming, bring about brains in our children which are small, which have thinner cortex, which have less enzyme activity, which have fewer glial cells, fewer neurons, small neuronal cell bodies and brains which are less efficient. So, while it doesn't prove it, we can't afford to say that it's not true in man, and we'd better make the most of it for all of our children, and really for ourselves, too.

Vision, of course, as you well know, is the big source of input, the big source of our learning; vision not just the two eyeballs, but vision in this broad sense that you in optometry have come to think of vision. I think it is a beautiful diagram and a beautiful concept of vision as being equated with intelligence and with understanding, and taking into the picture every aspect of development. I think it's something that people in other disciplines can use. I make use of this all the time in talking to mothers and fathers of newborn babies in showing them what they can do to help prevent some of these problems.

I would like to take just a minute or so and go through what I say and do in the use of these four circles. I understand there are some educators and psychologists and representatives of other disciplines here who may not have had any exposure to this. I'd be interested, also, to hear from some of the optometrists, and Dr. A.M. Skeffington maybe particularly since this whole thing originated with him, about my idea of this. If any of you would have any further suggestions about how this might be useful in working with parents in helping them explain the nature of their child in what they might need. And of course, there are the two circles representing the developing child. With him, we have the four overlapping circles, Circle A, B, C, and D. With A being Antigravity processes or locomotion. And of course, all of these are going on at the same time and reinforcing one another. But the baby circles first and then he scoots backwards and forwards, he crawls, he creeps, he walks around his environment, he hops and skips and jumps.

Circle B is Centering processes or location. One day the baby's hand comes up in front of him and he centers on it visually. He locates it, then he locates his error one, then he realizes they're his and he has some control over them. With a little thought, we can see where these two reinforce one another. Let's say for example, you put the bat down on the floor and he sees something interesting over there and it stimulates him to move. He goes over there and examines that with all of his senses. Because he's moved over there, he can now center on something else visually down there. He locates that. So, having moved, he locates more and the more he locates, the more he moves, et cetera.

Circle C is Identification processes or labeling. He hears his parents and others about him speaking to one another and at various objects and in his own mind, even in his early infancy, he's hooking labels onto things. And of course the more objects he's located, the more things he has labels on. The more new terms, the more new labels he hears—and he says, "Now what's that? Where's that?" the more that stimulates him to locate. And the more he locates the more he moves, the more he locates the more he labels.

You get to Circle D, communication processes or language, and he now begins to speak these labels he's learned. He speaks verbs and pronouns and communicates his desires and communicates not only verbally but in many other ways—body language, so called. He communicates with facial expressions and all sorts of things that all of us are communicating with all the time without our realizing it. Have you seen this book, *Body Language*? It's really a very interesting subject. The more labels the child has, the more language he's going to have. All these things then are reinforcing one another. Since these are all reinforcing one another, therefore mobility, locomotion and language are reinforcing one another.

In the center we have E, the emergent, which is a part of all of these. This emergent, then, is vision in its broad sense. This is intelligence and this is understanding. What is the teacher working on in school? The average teacher, of course, is working on C and D, labeling and language. If this child has significantly missed out down here in his infancy in antigravity and centering processes, if he in this spiral of development—if down here, some of these particular types of inputs are missing, from Circle A and Circle B, they're still missing up here. This could be the hyperactive child with the reading problem and the functional visual problem that we discussed before. So, if you're going to do anything about it, you have to go back down and start over again in the four circles, resupply the missing links, redevelop and reorganize him and bring him back up to the more efficient levels of operating.

Then, of course, all of this has a lot to do with eyeball vision, too, with sight, with development of convergence, development in fusion, development of binocularity, moving the eyes in a coordinated way, in helping him to develop vision in this broad sense. I don't have to tell you how many children have been said to have normal vision, and they don't see the world at all as it is down here.

I really like this diagram and all of the implications in it. Parents see it and go along with it completely, so there's no problem at all about getting them to put the children down on the floor and give them these opportunities.

At this time we will go into a little bit of what we do as far as diagnosis is concerned and treatment and how it relates to what you are all doing and how we are working together with developmental optometrists and people from various other disciplines. First of all, as in any situation, it is essential to get an accurate history and you're all involved in getting histories, too. I know in medicine it's considered that the diagnosis can be made at least 75% of the time by asking the right questions, without ever examining a patient or doing a test or anything. If you ask the right questions and get accurate answers, you know what's wrong with the patient 75% of the time. So that, of course, is the first thing. In this regard, we are looking for some particular items, such as the prenatal and the natal history, what happened around the time he was born—pregnancy, labor, delivery, was he premature, was it a difficult delivery. In other words, looking for some incident that might have happened that would lead to a brain injury. There are many more newborn babies who are brain-injured than we think.

There've been some studies done in which they did spinal taps on all the babies that came into the nursery which establishes criteria for brain injury, obvious brain injury, also blood and spinal fluid and increased spinal fluid pressure. They found that up to 75% of the babies met one or more of these criteria. Most of them, of course, looked normal, they acted normally, they ate as they should and there was nothing apparent. But maybe some of the children that you see and that we see the hyperactive child with all these symptoms,- might be one of those 75%, who suffered some unsuspected injury at the time he was born, just being born from what we consider a normal, ordinary labor and delivery. It may not be as normal as we think.

And then of course we go into the developmental milestones. Particularly, did this baby have opportunity in infancy to move? Was he restricted in infancy? Was he immobilized on his back, or was he in a jump seat, a swing seat, a walker, a play pen or something that didn't give him opportunity for these antigravity activities? Opportunities to spend sufficient time in these low mobility levels. When did he walk? When or did he crawl and if so what type of pattern did he crawl with and did he crawl on his stomach? Did he creep? When did speech start, and various other aspects concerning all these things. What about illnesses? Did he have long, persistent, very high fevers? What about accidents, particularly head injuries?

Was there any period of unconsciousness? How about his feeding history—chewing and sucking and swallowing as a newborn baby? What foods did he eat? What foods is he eating now? Might there be some indication of malnutrition as being a part of it? What about allergies? Does he have any known allergy? This could also be a very significant factor. And of course the family history—mother and father, are they living, are they well? What about siblings and their ages and what about their situation? Is there any such thing as diabetes in the family? And while this may not seem to be directly related to the whole area of functional visual problems and learning disabilities, still we're finding more and more that a history of diabetes in the family is a significant factor. As we'll mention a little later on, we've been looking at some of the metabolic aspects of the problem, including checking a five-hour glucose tolerance test and we find that a high percentage of children with this problem, that is, with learning disabilities, also have an abnormal glucose tolerance test. We must have about at least 85 now, I guess, and out of the 85 there are probably no more than 20 to 25 that fall into what is generally considered to be a normal glucose tolerance curve.

So, diabetes is an essential bit of information, because the incidence of an abnormal glucose tolerance curve in children is higher in those children in whom there is a history of diabetes in the family. You all know the relationship to the incidence of functional visual problems and learning problems, and so that's related too. Also we need to know the educational history. How did he do in kindergarten, first grade and second—whatever grade he's in? What about his reading and math? In other words, we need to go into every aspect of this medical and educational history that might give you a clue as to the cause of the problem and therefore give you some clues as to some of the specifics as to what to do about the problems.

Then we do the physical examination—just to be sure that there isn't some obvious physical problem that may have been unsuspected, too, which may be a significant factor in the school problem. We do a neurological examination which includes checking for and watching his gait. How does he stand? Can he stand with his feet together and arms down and eyes closed, or does he lose his balance when he does that? We check his sensory modalities—pain and light touch and hot and cold. We check all of his motor aspects—the movement, the strength, the tone of all his muscles. Is there tightness of heel cords or adductor muscles? Checking his cranial nerves, checking his reflexes and some tests of cerebella function—the old finger-to-nose test and finger-to-finger which I think you include in your developmental visual analysis.

And then we go into various laboratory tests—the complete blood count and urinalysis—the current one, not one that was done 6 mos. or a year ago. The five-hour glucose tolerance test, and one of those same specimens you can get at PBI—thyroid function. And also some of the radioactive uptake tests of thyroid function. An EEG. One might say, "Well, why bother with an EEG.?" Well, it's amazing sometimes at some of the things that sometimes turn up. It's true, most of the time, the EEG is normal, but there was an example just recently of a child with this whole symptom complex who didn't have any history of seizures and you really wouldn't suspect that you'd find anything on EEG but it came back with an abnormal report and the type of a tracing that could be caused from a cyst or a tumor or something on one side of the brain. There is low clinical evidence of it. So, this particular boy is scheduled for an encephalogram to see if there is something in there. So this is just one example of how checking into some of these things can turn up some information which is essential if any given treatment program is going to be effective.

Then we look at the trace minerals. More and more we're finding that probably a fair number of us in the room have a trace mineral imbalance. How do you find out about that? You could get a blood specimen and check for sodium, potassium, copper, cadmium, magnesium, manganese, iron and so forth, but that won't tell you what the situation is in the tissues or in the cells. But there is a readily available source of this and that is the sample of hair; hair being representative of the situation in other tissues in the cells. There is a Dr. John Miller, a biochemist in West Chicago who has been looking into this for a number of years and getting the ratios of each one of these to each other one. He has come up now with a tendency to find certain ratios in certain conditions. There are mineral supplements available to reestablish the proper mineral balance. If there is a significant imbalance here nutritionally, you could be way off and the visual training or whatever program he's on may not be effective at all. The glucose tolerance is also important; the feeling is more and more something we should look into. One of the symptoms that these kids show, for example, who have an abnormal glucose tolerance curve—there may be dizziness, there may be headache, there may be abdominal pain. They may be going along very well during the early part of the day and then around 11 o'clock they just go to pieces. Or it may be chronic fatigue, or fatiguing very easily. Is there anybody here who says, "That's me?" It could be. There are probably more adults with this type of thing than we realize.

There's an example of one boy who was in the Montessori school and he would go along beautifully—start school at 9 o'clock and he'd just go very well until about 11 o'clock, and then he would just go berserk. He'd start throwing materials and they just couldn't do anything with him. They looked into this with him and here the curve started up in a normal way and started down in a normal way, but then you got out to the three and four-hour interval and the bottom just dropped out of his blood sugar. So in this case, you put him on a low carbohydrate, high protein, and a frequent feeding diet. It was amazing the change that came about in him, just from changing his diet. So, he's just one of a number who are out there; not that this is the whole answer to the problem by any means, but nutrition is something that we are in medicine really neglecting. We talk about nutrition, but very often it's more lip-service than anything else.

Audiology—are these children hearing as they should be hearing things? Not that they have a gross hearing deficit, but they just may not be getting things in as they should be. We need to do a psychological evaluation, not just for IQ but for various other items of information that can come out of psychological evaluations, doing such tests as the WISC, the Peabody, Merrill Palmer, and the Bender-Gestalt. We're thinking now, too, of maybe at least in some instances doing the Rorschach on some of these. You wonder in interpreting a Rorschach whether you're really getting what you think you are. If an individual has a functional visual problem, then he's not even seeing the whole block of ink at one time. So there may be some correlation between their results on the Rorschach and vision. It's rather an interesting thing to think of.

A very important part of the evaluation is the developmental visual analysis. We've been working with several developmental optometrists in the Chicago area—I'm sure some of you know Drs. Ed Kasperek, Bob Johnson and Henry Moore. It was really through them that we became aware of the whole idea of developmental vision.

Then an evaluation of neurological organization as it relates to some of the details of these lower mobility levels is done looking at the details of crawling, creeping, hopping, skipping, jumping, and all those things. In addition also, part of this is checking for cerebral dominance. We still a lot we have to learn about dominance, too of course. As in this whole field, we're still really in a very primitive state of knowledge about the brain and how it works and how we learn. There is also educational testing, the reading tests, for example, just to mention one. Of course, there are whole numbers of possibilities in the educational testing line.

Once we gather all of this information through the developmental optometrist, the psychologist and so forth, then what do you do about it? I'd like to say something about what we are doing with many of the children. In forcing the usual learning situation on a neurologically disorganized child is a fine way to destroy teacher, home and child. These children need an intensive, positive, therapeutic developmental program which will build their self-confidence by improving motor coordination and visual auditory motor integration. For them, the time spent not learning in the classroom, lessening their self-esteem just adds to the obstacles we are trying to overcome. They need to get out of the classroom for a part of the day and into the gym where they will have opportunity to develop a good foundation in motor skills and motor patterns on which to build higher level perceptual and targeted skills. For the past eight years now at the Chicago Center, we've been teaching parents what to do with these children on an individual home program of motor activities that includes crawling, creeping, and some visual exercises and so forth. But we were finding children who we really weren't making it with and we were beginning to think that these were children who needed some of what you are doing in developmental optometry. During this time, we had not been communicating with the developmental optometrist.

On the other hand, they were seeing some children whom they were beginning to think needed some of what we were doing. We were both beginning to believe that physical education played an important part here. Not just getting the kids out playing games but developmental physical education; physical education as it relates to the learning process—basic movement education. Really, this is the key to education—the key to education is the developmental physical education. To help build in these lower level automatic activities. There was a man in Chicago, who unfortunately has gone back East, who was coordinator of physical education at a local YMCA. He had become interested in movement education, studied in Germany under Dr. Diem who has spent her life in this. He came back to Chicago and was beginning to put some of these developmental programs into the YMCA's, even the so-called Diaper Gym and Swim Programs. But he was having a little trouble with some of his instructors, getting them to see what he was talking about. So he was looking for somebody like us in other disciplines to sort of reinforce what he was saying. We were looking for somebody like him in physical education who thought developmentally about physical education as we were beginning to think about it. So we met accidentally and really through some of us having some children in some of these Diaper Gym and Swim Programs. The outcome of it was that we put together this combination of approaches that we'll have a little bit more to say about here in a minute. These things then have been applied for the prevention as well as the treatment of reading and learning difficulties.

To the groups that we're talking about, the individuals that we're talking about, I say we work with developmental optometrists. We really work very closely with them, to the point where some of them have actually had some of their staff come to the Center and work with the children who are on the group visual motor integration program in bringing some of the more advanced visual training to those children in the group program who were ready for it. And of course, this was all designed and prescribed by the optometrists who also then saw the children in their office and followed up on them as far as what has happened with them. Now more recently, we're working even more closely together. Previous to just the last few weeks, when I would see one of these children, it would be in the outpatient department of Loyola University Hospital or of another hospital. This came about because as time went on at the Chicago Center, we got so busy with all these children—for a period of time, I was full-time Medical Director at the Center, and then gradually for a variety of reasons, came back into doing general pediatrics as well as working with these children. But we were sending them all over Chicago, from Skokie—those of you who are familiar with Chicago, way up on the north side—to Ed Kasperek on the south side, to Loyola University Hospital on the west side. It really got to be quite a problem with some.

So now, since Dr. Vittenson, the psychologist, the optometrists, the audiologists have been communicating, getting together and teaching one another, we now have in the office the facilities for doing these. So the audiologist and the psychologist come, and sometimes one of the developmental optometrists are there at the same time. We have the facilities right there at one location, in the office, for them to come when I'm not there in pediatrics, and do these developmental evaluations, so that we have an even more coordinated multidisciplinary evaluation. When Dr, Vittenson does a psychological evaluation, she's doing it knowing what I do and what the optometrists do and what the audiologist does and vice versa, so that we also eliminate duplication. If one does, say, a test of auditory discrimination, there's no use for the other one to do it, which formerly was the case. So you see, we are working very closely together. This is not necessarily in the same way, but the idea of persons in various disciplines cooperating and learning from one another and utilizing the information that each has is what is necessary really to do right by the kids with these problems.

What does the treatment consist of? Of course, there is a whole variety of different things, depending on the child's particular problem. On the basis of all of these evaluations, specific needs may be met and the staff will know more exactly what one particular child requires in his treatment program. Some children, for example, require special training lenses in order to ease the stress of near point school work while they are progressing on the individual home program that has been outlined for them. These would, of course, be prescribed by their developmental optometrist. Some may need only visual training. Some have a level of neurological organization that they don't need some of the crawling and the creeping part of it, so they would be getting just the visual training in the office of the optometrist. And, most of the time also, on some sort of a home program

There is great evidence that one factor—and we've talked about this before in a way—that one factor in neurological problems of all types is a chemical imbalance involving various enzyme systems, and insufficient amounts of various vitamins, particularly the D vitamins; also Vitamin C, Vitamin B and some of the essential amino acids. Dr. Linus Pauling, that you no doubt have heard of, was the one who really first started talking about this aspect of the problem. Ortho-molecular medicine as it's called. We have found that by giving, like many others before us, that by giving some children large doses of these vitamins—this is the so-called megavitamin therapy or the ortho-molecular treatment—which we can create an optimal molecular environment in their brain which in turn enables them to function in a more normal way.

More and more we're finding, as I mentioned before, that a high percentage have an abnormal glucose tolerance curve. These are the sugars that require insulin for their metabolism. One might say, "Well, gee, if his blood sugar is down, let's give him sugar and bring it up." But it doesn't work that way. That's the worst thing you can do, and some of these kids have a tremendous craving for sweets, and it's the worst thing. Because what happens, they ingest sugar, then the blood sugar starts going up, this stimulates the pancreas, and out comes a big shot of insulin and drops it down. In some, when the blood sugar comes down, the insulin pulls back sugar starts up again, out comes another shot. So they get an up and down curve. Their blood sugar is fluctuating all over the place. Some of them never do go up. For those of you not familiar with the glucose tolerance, you get a fasting blood sugar, then a small glucose solution, and then the blood sugar is checked, 30 min. later, one hour, two, three, four, five hours later. Normally, it will rise and peak in an hour and then by two hours. Then there's a range—it comes down to a fasting level, and then sort of levels off. But in these kids, you get this up and down sometimes, or maybe it doesn't rise very much at all, it will go up just a few points at half an hour, peak there, and then level off, the so-called flat curve. Or maybe it will come up and start down in a normal way and then like this one boy I talked about, drop way off down in three or four hours. Or maybe it will go up and precipitously drop off. And of course, giving sugar is just going to aggravate the situation. So you have to cut down on those sugars in the diet that require insulin for their metabolism.

Some may need, as I mentioned, a mineral supplementation based on the hair analysis. While the group visual motor integration program is a group program, still it is an individualized program in which considerable attention is given to each child and to his particular needs. The staff is trained to try to sense what this child's needs are at this moment and to try to supply it. They are also trained to think- -or to never think of a child as having a behavior problem. You know, "Oh, that kid that acts up all the time." But here's a child with a problem, an organic problem of disorganization and rather than condemn him for what he's doing, to ask why he is doing it and what do I have to do at this moment and tomorrow and the next day to help them alleviate it. The home programs that are outlined consist of some crawling, some creeping, walking the balance beam, various motor programs like that, plus some of the eye-tracking movements and so forth. Some of these are on a program with some of the optometrists, some aren't. It depends on their circumstances, too, as to where they live, for example, what would be more feasible.

The group program that we've alluded to so often the visual motor integration program. This treatment approach is an integration of motor coordination program for neurological organization with the developmental visual approach to the problem, the developmental physical education program of movement exploration, developed by Dr. Diem in Germany, together with a developmental swimming program and a program of rhythm instruction developed by Dr. Carl Orff.[4] Some of you no doubt are familiar with the Orff approach to teaching music to young children. We've had this going in the Montessori school for a number of years and have integrated that rhythm section of it into this program. Other activities and exercises draw extensively from the ideas of Kephart, Barsch, Harmon,

---

4. *From Wikipedia: Carl Orff (July 10, 1895 – March 29, 1982) was a 20th-century German composer, best known for his cantata Carmina Burana (1937). In addition to his career as a composer, Orff developed an influential method of music education for children.*

Montessori and others well known in the field of learning disabilities.

Children attend four days each week for one hour and 45 minutes daily for a 12-week session. Classes are small, maximum eight, and are supervised by a trained instructor plus two assistants. Children are placed in classes according to their ages and most of them from 8 to 12 with a few younger and a few up to maybe 16. And also they're grouped according to their level of neurological organization. The mobility aspect of it, the Doman-Delacato mobility program of neurological organization consists of providing children with an opportunity to duplicate normal development by repeatedly going through—going around a room entailing crawling in prone position, creeping, cross-pattern walking, as well as performing some of the in-between stages—so-called elephant walk, walking on their hands and feet. It's not intended to be simply physical exercise but it's a way of programming these basic movements into the neural system. These children would have performed these activities sufficiently if it were not for lack of opportunity, injury or disinherited developmental pattern. Some of these kids are at a somewhat lower level and require, prior to some of this mobility activity, actually patterning some of these movements into them; sort of priming the pump, you might say. In some cases, too, they go through a stylized type of training where the refinements of these movements are taught and accentuated by the child. This depends on the developmental level again of each one and the length of time that is spent in the program.

Approximately 30 minutes each day are spent in the mobility part of this. The equipment is very simple. The floor is covered with linoleum and carpet to give different types of tactile experiences. Harmon Boards are for balance walking and comprise another part of it.

Vision: The developmental visual program, of course as you well know, is an approach to the achievement of learning disabilities used by developmental optometrists. Here it is used as part of the overall treatment program. Each child progresses from low level visual activities on up through the higher cortical of visual exercises. Activities may begin with deep breathing and relaxation exercises and progress up through the various levels of eye-tracking movement, for example. Gross body movements are brought into play. For those of you in developmental vision, of course, you are well familiar with what this consists of. Part of it consists of, for those of you who aren't familiar with it, the use of vision training instruments as well as prisms and lenses under the direction of the consultant developmental optometrist to develop convergence, fusion, accommodation, depth perception, binocularity, good spatial relationships, and overall visual efficiency.

Rhythm: The rhythm program is implemented because we see the children, and I'm sure you've noticed this very often too, completely lack rhythm which is so essential for really all of our functioning. The whole universe is rhythm; speech is rhythm. And without it, we're just not going to function efficiently. By repeatedly listening to the rhythm created by the instructor and observing the rhythmic movements in making an attempt to imitate them, the child gradually begins to become aware of rhythm and begins to develop it. This is true not only in the rhythm class as such, but he also begins to use it in other areas of the program. As improvements are seen in the rhythm class, they're also seen in mobility; in the gym and also in swimming. When he has begun to develop visual and auditory memory and the ability to repeat rhythm, a child is given an opportunity to create his own rhythm which the class will then follow. In other words, for a short period of time, each child becomes the instructor of the class and this, over a period of time, greatly improves his self image and confidence through repeated successes at his own level. This whole thing follows Montessori principles, one of which is, never let a child just fail here until he's had a reasonable chance for success. It gives him many opportunities for successful experiences rather than a series of failures, which has been his lot usually up until this time.

In the developmental physical education program, as we said, it's based on the work of Dr. Diem. This concept of physical education is different from that which involves having the children play games only; games which presuppose that they have the basic physical development and the basic automatic movements which are laid down in infancy in the nervous system. Many children in physical education classes are forced to play games for which they are completely unfitted neurologically. And of course, what does this do? It adds to their failure. Because of this basic in-coordination, many do not take part in games on the playground or they do so reluctantly and often with great embarrassment and frustration. They can only take so much of this, so what's the next thing? Go into the house, sit down in front of the two-dimensional television set and just reinforce the problem by inactivity. Movement education or developmental gym gives a child opportunity to develop the proper neurological circuitry that he needs and to learn the basic movements which are essential to the learning process. Each child is allowed to function at his own level and in his own way. There is no competition between the children. For example, if ball activity is going on, each one has a ball. Each one does it in his own way, and for him, this is success.

Another thing that has many applications is a wand as it's called. Really, it's a sort of a painted, sawed-off broomstick. One of the things the instructor might say is, "Let's see who can balance it. Let's see how many different ways you can balance this Stick." So he will maybe do it on his hand. Some other kids will do it that way. Some will do it on their finger. Some more advanced will put it on their chin. But nobody's paying any attention to them. For him, he's balancing it, too. For him, it's success. And then as he develops in all these areas, he moves on to where he can do it like that, too, but nobody's paying any attention to the way he's doing it, they're too involved in their own.

Each child is given instructions on the trampoline and usually progresses from simple up-and-down jumping to performing some fairly complicated combinations of knee drops, front drops, sit drops and back drops in a variety of ways. The trampoline is a particularly useful piece of equipment for these children, inasmuch as it repeatedly and quickly takes a child from low brain levels to higher brain levels and back again. As he goes up in the air from the trampoline neurologically, he is functioning at a lower level. The higher he goes, the lower he comes down neurologically. Then he is given, in time, some cortical task to perform at the same time, such as counting backwards to complicate it a little bit. Or spelling a word, or otherwise using his cortex in some way. The various procedures followed in the gym as well as in other areas help a child to develop proper spatial relationships and to accurately realize the relationship of himself and his body parts to the space around him. This is something you see all the time in these kids who don't know whether they're up or down, before or behind or what.

Developmental swimming is a carefully structured developmental sequence with various children in different ability and developmental levels, divided into several groups. It transfers the benefits derived from mobility, vision, rhythm and gym activities to the medium of water. As a child improves in his crawling in a prone position, for example, a change is noted for the better in how he kicks while swimming and how he can now go in a straight line in swimming where previously he just couldn't kick or go at all. As his swimming improves, his self image and his self confidence improve. Swimming is sort of—you have to know how to do it if you're going to be one of the group. One can easily see how all areas of the program can reinforce each other.

The key to making a program such as this a successful one is, of course, the staff. The equipment is simple and the curriculum is somewhat limited by the specificity of each child's problems. Because we are concerned with learning processes rather than content the staff must be well trained as educational therapists capable of making on-the-spot evaluations of all areas. It's an on-going evaluation. Levels of neurological functioning must be well grounded in the cybernetic model of the learning processes. In addition, they must be capable of understanding the diagnostic concepts and carrying out treatment procedures of the various fields involved in this multidisciplinary type of treatment.

We mentioned the various fields, various disciplines that we're working with. Just to go through them, we have John Bassler. I think some of you have met him before—he's an educator in reading. There's a chiropractor who, strange as it might seem—it really isn't strange, but I mean as far as the medical profession and how they look on this—but they have something also to offer. Robert Cienkus is an M.A. and a Ph.D. candidate in reading. Robert Freeman, developmental has a Masters in Physical Education. Robert Johnson, O.D. and Kasperek, O.D. and Henry Moore, O.D. are optometrists in developmental optometry. Charles Muir, Masters and a Ph.D. candidate in reading and neurological organization. Susanne Van Nolde is a Masters with a Ph.D. candidate in reading. Lucya Prince, a Masters in rhythm, who does the music—or rather, who does the rhythm part. And Dr. Vittenson, the psychologist. There are also various others in some of the medical specialties that we call on at times—neurosurgeons. In other words, all the various specialties in medicine and optometry and all those in the child profession are represented.

Mobility: There are some examples from some of the optometrists who have been working with some of the children in vision training programs, and really not making the results that they felt they should be. They get them into more—and their home program didn't consist of any of the crawling and creeping and so forth. When they get into this type of program and then go back to their office again after a period of time. We had a call recently from Dr. Kasperek who was just amazed at the changes that took place in a patient of his after getting down to some of these more basic levels. There are those children who really probably are not ready for regular vision training until they get organized at some of these lower automatic levels.

There's a very important part of all of this in view of all of our dealings with anybody, and that is the old positive mental attitude. You get into the whole field of parapsychology which could be a subject for a whole session, but the image that we have of ourselves first of all in doing this, and the image that you have of yourselves in your work, and the image that we have in our own subconscious that we may not even realize, the image that we have of the child we're working with is extremely important in whether or not we are successful with them. Because the image that we have is the image that we project, and these kids have tremendous intuition. They really know what we're thinking, and the image that we project is the one that they receive and the one that they react to. So what we project is what we get back. We're all transmitting and receiving all the time, and just like a radio, what it pulls in over the antenna is what comes out the speaker. The same thing is true of these kids. So it behooves us and the parents—and here's where we can help educate the parents—to try to get them to develop a positive image, to develop an actual visual picture of this child being able to do and to be what we would all like him to be. By doing that, we've taken a big step forward in helping him to achieve what might be possible for him.

I'd just like to summarize by saying that the neurological, well-organized child with good vision in this broad sense of the word, teaches himself. The knowledge of how to prevent and correct many of the physical causes of reading and learning difficulties and of the functional visual problems and superimposed emotional problems already exists. It exists in the various specialty disciplines of medicine, optometry, psychology, education, nutrition and every other related discipline. But it is yet to be fully integrated and applied. Efforts must continually be made to educate, particularly the students in these disciplines and particularly, I would say, medical students. The optometry students are being educated along this way, but particularly to educate medical students and the present practicing doctors, too, but it's easier to reach the students, regarding these concepts. Optometrists individually, as I'm sure you're already doing, should take every opportunity to acquaint physicians and especially those dealing with children with what you do and try to foster a cooperating, working arrangement with them. Now I know in some cases this is not an easy thing to do, but gradually, at least keeping it in mind, and gradually working out I think in time this education of the various professions involved will come about. One example where the physicians working with you could be of great help is in the metabolic aspects and getting some of the testing—the glucose tolerance and so forth. How, knowing doctors, knowing physicians, it wouldn't go over very big for an optometrist to say to him, "I want this child to have a glucose tolerance test." You can see the reaction you might get sometimes. But if we get this pulling together and pooling of knowledge, there wouldn't be that much of a problem. You as optometrists have a great opportunity in working with families to educate parents regarding their infants and young children, and what they can do with their children at this age to help foster and train good vision in this broad sense, and good neurological organization, and prevent the development of these very significant problems that really constitute one of the biggest problems in the whole pediatric age group in this country. It really is one of the biggest public health problems we have—the whole area of learning disabilities.

In some schools, it is 75, 80, or even 90% of the children who have it. Functional visual problems, you'll find, probably in 100% of them. In your home programs with children who already have problems, having established rapport with them through working with the child with a problem but also talking to them about their normal children and about normal development and the needs of normal children, you can more readily then possibly institute some of these mobility programs at lower levels. Some of the crawling and creeping, for example, of the development, some of these low-level aspects which, from my experience, may well make your vision training programs even more effective than they already are; those kids who can benefit from vision training if they also have these low-level automatic activities for them so that they don't have to use their cortical energy down at the level that should be automatic, so that they can now use their cortex for these higher intellectual functions and enable them to work efficiently.

Only through this educational process and through fearless dedicated cooperation of all of us in the child profession, will we enable all children to function at peak effort of sufficiency and to achieve their true potential. Thank you very much.

Ray Wunderlich, MD (Pediatrician)
A Pediatric Look at the Mal-adapting Child
1972

One of the points I have repeated with my optometric friends is what you are doing appears to be a form of a neurological examination of the human organism. But when I see optometrists observing motor behavior and doing the refined analysis of function, I cannot escape the fact, you are doing functional neurology -- and I hope that gives your egos a boost the next time you're talking with your friendly neurologist.

I would like to talk about neurological function because I think it's intimately related to what optometry does. I'd like to reiterate we learn from the abnormal and then we apply it to the normal. We learn, for instance in medicine, from diseased states. This is the way that medicine has developed, from a pathology-oriented discipline to one which can begin to turn its attention to function; for example, the vitamin deficiency diseases are well known to optometry. Columbus's sailors sucked on limes so they wouldn't get scurvy. Rickets, beriberi, pellagra are all examples of disease entities due to vitamin deficiencies. The appreciation of these disorders led to an appreciation of the importance of the vitamin in health. We now know that there are at least some 30 vitamin-dependency diseases in which the need or requirement for a particular vitamin exceeds the normal daily requirement for most of us. So this has led us to consider what is optimal for each individual versus merely adequate.

Another example is with mentally handicapped individuals. In this group, we know that 10 to 25% of these individuals are severely handicapped --if you look at the population. These individual have an organic, biological origin. That leaves the bulk of mentally handicapped individuals, making up some 75-90% of the group, who are educable. This group has been termed to be of social-cultural origin and to be mild. Therefore it is appropriate to think of normal human function in our society as biologically based, but predominantly derived from socio-cultural factors. Hunger, thirst, sex and sleep are the needs we all have that underlie our basic behavior. Next we could list aggression, violence, war, cooperation, competition, status, and indeed even problem solving, as biologically based but with a strong cultural origin. The main point is that man develops his brain function as well as his brain dysfunction by social organization and cultural traits as well as by nutrition and heredity.

The problem with the child in your office can be solved by and large by social manipulation and by altering the environment of the child, so that both must be attended to. This physiologic framework of the individual is what you're dealing with many times when you're watching the changes in the visual system. I say to you, "Why is the range like that, and why is it fixed and slow to become flexible?" We look to you for those answers.

I'd like to talk about the body and the mind as a continuum. I feel there is no dichotomy, so we'll talk about mind-body. It is the task of the brain to make sense out of the environment and ones' internal self. In order to do this well, a goal or purpose is necessary. It appears this is a frontal lobe function of the brain, and Alexander Luria[1] has given evidence of this. If there is no goal or purpose for the individual, if there is frontal lobe dysfunction, the individual dies in one sense or another. Some problem must be perceived in order for the organism to frontally set a goal for itself, and these perceived problems must appear to the organism to be attainable by virtue of some effort. Therefore we can view brain function or brain dysfunction, as a relative matter relative to the tasks presented to the organism in the environment, whether it's one of you reading a nearpoint chart or whether it's a kid trying to do what his teacher wants.

This calls your attention to the organic core of the onion, if you will, to the nucleus, to the germ of the matter with the environmental-social, interactional matters surrounding it. Various organic factors should be considered in the child including some to get you thinking. The amount of weight gained during pregnancy, for instance. I bet you have factors like this on your history forms, but what do you do about them? You don't do much because perhaps you're not aware of these factors. A pregnancy in which there is a weight gain of less

---
1. *Alexander Romanovich Luria (16 July 1902 – 14 August 1977) was a famous Soviet neuropsychologist and developmental psychologist. He was one of the founders of cultural-historical psychology and psychological activity theory.*

than some 15 pounds is suspect and is apt to produce a vulnerable child. The pattern of weight gain during a pregnancy is apt to be an important factor also. Does it occur in the first trimester or only later? The labor and delivery, of course, have been implicated for many years in the production of problems in children; the ranges of behavior and performance may be constricted or restricted. They may become preservative rather than nice flexible creatures, or they become excessively tight or loose individuals. We see excessively narrow births in which the labor is short; 1-2 hours, or excessively prolonged or dysfunctional. Space within the skull is considered just to point out that external space is not the only matter that is of importance, but the internal factors or spatial arrangements on a gross basis are important too. Are the skull sutures grown together so that the brain cannot grow? Is there a blood clot? Is there a hygroma of water or some other arrangement which is limiting mechanically the available growing of the brain which occurs kaleidoscopically in the first year or two of life? Are there circulatory problems? Are the blood vessels compressed and collapsed in a low blood pressure type of state secondary to nutritional and mineral factors? Are there blood vessel abnormalities, etc.? Are there hemorrhages and adhesions? Do the parents, grandparents, and relatives have reading problems?

This applies also to various neurological signs. I see families who have abnormal Babinski signs indicating abnormality in the cortico-pyramidal system. I see this in the families of these individuals. They may have no deficit at all in their society as much as they are stressed but they are carrying a neurological deficit which may never become apparent in their particular society. And so there are hereditary disturbances of brain dysfunction of limitation of abilities.

The chemical problems, of course, are many and varied. They include carbon monoxide exposures, lead intoxication, carbohydrate metabolism disorders, thyroid disturbances and many others. The matter of protein intake during the pregnancy and the early infancy of the child is quite crucial. We know that the woman who has a very poor nutritional protein intake during her pregnancy is apt to have toxemia or eclampsia and perhaps have abnormal placenta-fetal relationships, or pre-mature deliveries. We know the brain cells of animals and, presumably, humans cease to multiply around

6-9 months post-natally. This is dependent on the protein intake that the child has, therefore you do have a chance during the first year of life to add to your neurological stores if you have a proper nutritional intake with complete protein during that time period.

If we take a broad look at the nervous system, you can categorize it in various ways, but this is one way that I would suggest. It is not complete. The autonomic nervous system; you deal with every day in your practices with the visceral elements: the pupillary reflexes, the smooth muscles, and the behavioral changes that you see in the individual. He suddenly grows pale, sweats, faints, passes out, etc., or becomes constipated or has a bowel episode. The sympathetic nervous system and parasympathetic nervous system are nothing new to you. The spinal cord is concluded there.

The brain itself can be thought of in several groups. The first is the brain stem, the core of the brain in which the reticular activating system resides. The reticular activating system, spreading up like a fan all over the brain, is a widespread system which travels up from the lower brain stem to the cortex of the brain which serves to activate or energize multiple areas. It is here that there is a delicate balance in the system between excitations and inhibition. When you consider that some 50% of the brain's energy is devoted to inhibition, disrupting these, you can understand why some kids are hyperactive. These kids may have convulsions or random, disorganized behavior because of a failure of the inhibiting system. There are probably two bundles or two phases of this particular activating system, two functional systems anyway: the one inhibitory and the other excitatory. Here again, we have the critical balance. You must have certain areas excited so you can stay awake and write down things on the lecture paper, but to put your probes in the right way, you must inhibit other areas. If you observe children, and you consider this neurological disorganization that people have spoken about, then you can see the problems they have in balancing the stimulated areas and the inhibited areas. One name for these children who are neurologically deprived or deficient is the disinhibited child, disinhibited behavior. You will be hearing a great deal more about this area and the neuro-chemistry of this area in this decade.[2]

---

2. *Editor's Note: Here the author, as early as 1972, is predicted the epidemic of attention problems in children that will be seen far in the future and which continues to this day (2010).*

The rear part of the brain is the sensory part, the primary reception areas of the brain and the all-important association areas to which the primary receiving areas send out messages in order to derive the meaning of the primary reception areas. And this, of course is what makes us human. We have association areas in great abundance compared to lower animals. The frontal lobes, I have already talked about as the achievement-setting areas, which are necessary for the organism to be able to have a zestful, enthusiastic, motivating approach to the tasks that he perceives. The person who lacks this may have a problem in the frontal lobes.

The motor area is in the frontal lobes. Communication must occur between the two cerebral hemispheres. The right cerebral hemisphere is largely visual-spatial—that's space—and the left cerebral hemisphere is largely language or verbal and auditory. If you are going to have integration and matching of these and appreciation of differences of inputs, visual and auditory input for instance, one has to have communication within the brain just like one has to have communication within the classroom or office.

I'd like to read to you at this point a little note from the collaborative study of cerebral palsy which was carried on by the National Institute of Neurological Disease and Stroke. They surveyed over 55,000 deliveries in 14 of our leading medical centers finding a direct relationship between the weight gain in pregnancy, the birth weight, and neurological damage in the infant. Those mothers who had gained 36 pounds or more had about one-third the numbers of brain-damaged children as those who had gained 0 to 15 pounds. I punch this again because of the past dictum that has been law that you shouldn't gain too much weight. Here again we may ask: What is the optimal weight gain for this individual? Gradually the feeling has come about that perhaps the woman ought to set her own level within wider ranges than we have ever considered in the past.

I'd like you to think of the causes of these problems that prevent the child from achieving or giving you a normal visual profile. I'd like to have you think that it may be within the neurological system or within the chemical systems of the body because the chemical systems and the neurological systems are vastly interrelated.

If we look at brain dysfunction—and we call it dysfunction because that's what it is; it's not necessarily damage, there are those children who have damage; you can demonstrate damage. If a child has insufficient thyroid hormone in his blood, he doesn't grow very well; his bones don't grow. He has an abnormal electroencephalogram and he may function poorly in school. His vision may show as a problem in your office, so it behooves you to ask the question: Could this child have low thyroid function which depresses this organism and which is the cause of his visual dysfunction or a major contributing factor? The chemical causes of a dysfunctioning organism, brain, mind, body, are disordered fluids surrounding the neurons or nerve cells themselves. These disordered fluids surrounding the nerve cells -- I have just chosen the low thyroid hormone in the surrounding fluid as one example. A more common example would be the child with hypoglycemia. Naturally if there are toxins circulating within the body such as lead or some other toxic minerals: cadmium etc., this can stop the cellular metabolism of the neurons and the cells in the retina, etc., and give you a similar profile. Naturally these types of problems are often occurring. Here I have the situation where both of these are intact: the hardware is intact, and the fluid surrounding the hardware is intact in the nervous system but the environment, the external climate of the child is not sufficient to permit that social organization and social programming of the individual which gives him a normal achievement or satisfaction of goals. That viewpoint is one which is not static and not fixed. It is one which I feel applies. It is not the viewpoint of the neurologist who is more oriented to a fixed model.

The child we're talking about most often presents with the picture of the hyperactive child. The hyperactive child referred to you by the teacher because he is a wall climber, who then sits still in your office. What about this? You write a letter back and say, "This child isn't hyperactive. He didn't do a thing here. He was quite attentive." Is he hyperactive or isn't he? This completely ignores the matter of setting I pointed out earlier. Many of us are hyperactive under some circumstances. Our behavior changes under certain circumstances. Children with minimal neurological dysfunction may only be hyperactive under some probes, under some settings, and may be quite capable of not being hyperactive under other circumstances. It does not mean that the child does not have a problem of control of goal orientation of achievement. People are different. You must have a mirror before you if you're so lucky to find out what message you are telescoping to the child, to the "hyperactive child" in front of you. Perhaps you are sending a message which says, "Calm down. It is O.K. It's safe. I am in control. There is no fear. You can be still under these circumstances." Other personalities and behaviors telegraph the message to the child that there is a risk here and their nervous system does not turn off but remains excessively turned on.

The impulsive behavior, aggression, sometimes violence that you see in these children, is sometimes extreme. I remember a child who was destroying everything in sight. This was a 6-year old who was tearing up the beds, throwing the dishes down and destroying the lawn, flora and fauna. The family could barely control him at all. We treated that child with cortisone and we had an immediate response, within a few days, and we could titrate his degree of violence by the amount of cortico-steroid we gave him. Ritalin had no effect on this child and he had been seen in a number of child guidance clinics for several years with very little result. Again, this shows you the organic base of some behavior which can be altered under certain therapeutic situations; the language disorders, the incoordination, you're all quite aware of these better than I, perceptual disorders and so on.

Now I'd like to comment on the intellectual deviations. Here the children often exhibit high degrees of ability in some intellectual areas. Some of these children are absolute geniuses. There seems to be some correlation of high achievement on some intellectual test results with a change in neurological wiring. These children apparently are wired so that they can process information in some areas very well, thus they become almost idiot savants in some areas, but they usually process poorly in others. These are the areas that get them into trouble and bring them to our offices and to mine and to the psychological therapists.

The treatment of these children labeled minimal brain dysfunction is a question about where we start. I have seen visual training handle many of these children with neurological dysfunction who have clear-cut soft neurological signs and some had neurological signs. You do not know that because sometimes it is difficult to find this information if you do not have close medical communication. Behavioral counseling can alter the behavior, by affecting aspects in the stimulus response setup, and can do it very well by bringing to the family and the child an awareness of behavior. Remember, this behavior is often ruining families, causing divorces and testing parents and teachers to the limit. These are very, very serious problems and so perhaps you are seeing them on a lower level. Behavioral counseling can bring about immediate results; if the therapist is aware that all behavior has meaning and that all behavior can be shaped. The behavior can be shaped in two ways: 1) by ignoring the behavior, which is more standard and consistent with the psychological advice that you will probably be seeing, and 2) by not ignoring the behavior but by paying attention to it. There are some negative behaviors, unwanted behaviors, which must be ignored. There are some negative, unwanted behaviors that cannot be ignored. If one only believes that behavior modification should ignore the unwanted behavior only, he will have that many more failures. A good aversive stimulus sometimes is worth three months of ignoring the behavior.

The medical avenues of treatment for these children in a continuum are—the stimulant drugs. They've had quite a bit of prevalence in the press the last year or two, although they are quite safe in supervised hands. The danger in the use of the stimulants—such as Ritalin and amphetamines—is that they will be used and the symptoms will be pushed down to the level of tolerance which is great, but nothing else will be done.

Again I must say that these will be the parents, the job holders, and the drivers of tomorrow. I would urge for the long view in these individuals and for the investigations to show whether the problem areas have just now, with the use of stimulants, been made so they can be examined and looked at in a more calm and orderly fashion in a family inter-dynamic situation. The use of these drugs brings improvement in 70-75% of children. They should not be used indiscriminately. On the other hand, they should be used with supervision and feedback, hopefully, from vision specialists and therapists, and physicians communicating together.

The antihistamine drugs are very interesting. They are Benadryl or Dilantin,[3] and they are often responsible for favorable change in these children. I would like to know whether or not you find changes in the visual system when these drugs are being used. The anti-convulsants, Dilantin, Mebrerial or Mysoline, Petimalare, are an interesting group. On occasion even when there are no convulsions in a child, we use these as a therapeutic trial. When children have epileptic equivalents such as abdominal aches and pains on a cyclic basis, headaches, aggressive or violent behavior, it's just amazing how frequently one can get a result here also.

The anti-allergy treatments, which I'll go into later, use a specific chemical agent if it is found to be deficient. But, we often see multiple problems in the metabolic sphere when there is a chemical deficiency. For instance, the calcium may be low, the blood sugar may tend to be low, the thyroid hormone in the blood may tend to be low and the level of eosinophils, or blood cells in the peripheral blood count, is apt to be high, indicating some kind of metabolic disintegrity. Physical therapy, occupational therapy and other forms of motor therapy I find to be very important. Very often these children are so handicapped by their disabilities that they have had practically no exercise of a vigorous nature and I find them many times to have muscles of putty, hearts that race when you exercise inadequate cardiac reserve, and inadequate pulmonary reserve in breathing from the fact that they are not able to do very much in a consistent way.

The use of orthomolecular medicine in the form of mega-vitamins, particularly, with other mineral therapies is extremely important and probably will go far to replace the medical therapies that I have been covering. The common story is that of a hyperactive child; he cannot attend; he cannot focus his eyes, and then if we find no specific deficiency we can treat him with mega-vitamins and within a few months we find the child is losing the infections that he has. Many times his allergies are disappearing, his visual system is improving in its efficiency in the motor aspects of it and his processing of information is increasing concomitantly. The mega-vitamins are the high doses of "B" and "C" vitamins in very high doses and the effect is very mysterious. If any of you have problems this way yourselves, I

3. *Editor's Note: The medications in use have evolved and would now include many more such medications used for ADD and ADHD.*

would urge you to seek counsel regarding orthomolecular medicine because it is one of the best tools available to me in the handling of children with problems.

In my office, problems of adaptations, has been the administration of mega-vitamins to the parents. I had a patient from Palm Beach who had been everywhere with their child. The child, unfortunately, had a microcephaly—small head—with mental retardation. I couldn't help the child. However, I gave mega-vitamins to the parents and for the first time in their married life the mother and father were able to go to their friendly psychiatrist and accept counseling—and like it. And so these are tools we can use to make your job easier in visual therapy and perhaps even in visual diagnosis.

Regarding brain function of the child, at least in our culture, there are many physiological problems probably also relating to vision which serve as an organic base providing this child with all of these symptoms and mal-adaptations that drive teachers, parents and therapists nuts. These are often able to be helped with standard medical approach and the therapy of these children envision training, for instance or perceptual motor therapy can often be helped greatly by the administration of a standard approach, that is, family investigation, the use of stimulants, tranquilizers, and anti-histamines. But in addition to that, we have a new tool available to us which is the administration of mega-vitamins which is able to transform the biologic base and to alter the physiological problem sufficiently to give a new lease on life, a new grasp, a new achievement, motivation to these children. At this time the subgroups of these children has not been sufficiently identified so that we can predict which group of children will have the best results or require specific regimens. However, intense activity is now going on so that perhaps in another couple of years we will have more specific physiological therapy.

Allergies

We've heard a lot about allergies, and I'll talk about it, and you'll continue to read about it in the next 10 years because the science of immunology is having a rebirth and it is making great advances every year in understanding host resistance and what makes a host go wrong in regard to defense and regulation of the body, including the visual system.

The allergic problems we see on a clinical basis can be divided into two groups: First the obvious problems that everybody knows about: the kids who sneeze and wheeze, the ones who have hay fever, asthma, eczema, hives, etc. The extrinsic asthmatics are those who react to external particles in the environment, external antigens such as pollens, dust, mold spores and other particulate agents. The intrinsic asthmatics are the ones in which you can find practically no excitants which set off their systems. These individuals are postulated to have an inborn problem with the beta adrenergic system, the beta adrenergic receptors.

Allergy is an inappropriate reaction of the immune system. It means something is reacting in the way we would not expect it or want it to. Most likely a hyper-sensitive or allergic response is trying to rid the body of a foreign agent, and in so doing the system may be tripped off prematurely in some persons by virtue of hereditary traits or just by virtue of a tremendous overwhelming of the system due to a great number of particles bombarding It. And so we have the obvious symptoms and these can be called external systems because we can see a sneeze and hear a wheeze. These are releases of the system.

On the other hand less obvious allergic problems, hidden allergic problems, or the more subtle ones are probably ongoing and are completely unknown to the individual. These include low-grade sinus problems, post-nasal drip, perennial allergic rhinitis, some relation to vasomotor rhinitis. Illustrated by the child with a chronically congested or stuffy nose, the child who has recurrent, upper respiratory disorder, the child who has one cold after another or one cold which can't get well, the child with the allergic tension fatigue syndrome who is perhaps one day anxious, tense and hyper-excitable and perhaps the next day or later in the day when his energy has worn out is excessively fatigued and can't hack the material you're giving him or even to become personable in family or teacher relations.

Allergic tension fatigue syndrome produces neurological symptoms so that the child's brain is involved and he is either torpid or languid, or he is hyper-excitable, or impulsive and distractible. Perhaps the food that he has ingested either that morning or that day is causing his to act this way or possibly his system has been overwhelmed by particles in his environment such as an extra load of pollen, dust or some chemical excitant in the atmosphere. And so the hyper-active child is found many times to have an allergic basis for his problem. One of the clues we have is by looking at the blood count and seeing the number of "allergy cells" in the blood count. On a simple blood smear, if the technician upon examination sees these crazy looking cells that have red granules in them called eosinophils, a marker of the allergic state, and if these are significantly elevated, one can be fairly sure that an allergic problem exists. The normal range of these eosinophils, is perhaps 1-2% of the white blood cells on the differential white count. In the allergic state eosinophils are elevated 5, 10, 15, or even 20%, and so this simple test can be a marker if it is performed. Often it is not performed and the clue is missed. Eosinophilscan also be elevated in the presence of worms and certain other disorders, etc., but by and large we have eosinophilia in the presence of the allergic state.

During the first months of life we see babies with colic and indigestion who are giving their parents fits, and so we have the nucleus, the germ, of a problem established in the home. Because parents are only people, they, like the rest of us get shook and they over- or under-react, and so they can funnel in added emotional deprivation and over stimulation problems to the child who is demanding some response. This is often the case with the child who appears to have colic, who is giving his parents a hard time, especially going to sleep at night, and who very often has allergy of one form or another. Oftentimes these children are allergic to milk, maybe hypersensitive to something in the mother's breast milk, or they may be swallowing a good deal of mucous that is coming down from their nose or small sinuses and having an allergy from the environmental air they are breathing. Some of these children we have helped a great deal by changing milk. Often it will not work and one has to think then of the air the child is breathing and often we have helped these children by having them breathe some kind of filtered air.

The child that we see who has his tonsils and adenoids removed is another child that most commonly is found to have some kind of immune or allergic problem to account for the increase in the lymph tissue in the tonsil and adenoid area. The younger the tonsils and adenoids are removed, the more likely that child is to have a definite or allergic or hypersensitivity problem. The dictum is that; if it is below three years of age, this child is an allergic child until proven otherwise.

I was told about a case in which the person had a tonsillectomy at a young age, and then a couple of years later had another tonsillectomy. This is a clear indication that something is in the system stimulating lymph tissue for regrowth because when you surgically whack something out and a couple of years later it is back again, there is some continuing hyper-stimulus or hyper-reaction on the part of that lymph tissue, which is making it become a growth structure again and apparently needed to be cut out. And so the regrown tonsils and lymph tissues are another indicator of the presence of a definite allergic problem that is making the tissue regrow. In the same individual who had the tonsil and adenoid regrowth, they had another two-year interval and the child had their appendix out. The appendix is a lymphoid organ; it has lymphoid tissue within it. And so you see there was some insult or hyper-reaction on the part of the lymph system in this individual. The fascinating thing is that as you go on and follow the life of this individual, you find that she has become hypoglycemic. She has a low blood sugar and has struggled with that in her mature adult life. One begins to wonder about the relationship of these problems in the host metabolism. We do find a high correlation between allergic problems and hyper-insulinism resulting in low blood sugar. Exactly what the relationship is, we do not know, but it's possible we have one problem on a continuing basis manifesting itself in different ways at different times.

The days when growing pains were just passed off are gone since there is usually some explanation for children with growing pains. In my experience these are often due to the ingestion of certain foods. Children react with leg aches at night or with the presence of a low-grade inflammation and low-grade infection secondary to allergy. Infection is often precipitated by the presence of a low-grade allergic state in the mucous membrane which lowers the integrity of the mucous membrane and allows the balance between host and bacteria to be tipped in favor of the bacteria.

The child with joint symptoms—aches and pains—may have rheumatic fever which, incidentally, is an allergic disease, hypersensitive to these symptoms due to a reaction of the host to streptococci bacteria. And so you see the great scope of the immune or allergic process operating in many of us and at times coming out as definable entities such as rheumatic fever, other times being more diffuse like joint pains, muscle ache, rheumatic-like pains, etc.

The child with nose bleeds is usually an allergic child. If it's 90 in your room, then you can dry out your nasal secretions and maybe pick them a little bit and get some bleeding, or you can get hit in the nose or you can have a tumor in the nose, etc., but 9 times out of 10 the kid with nose bleeds has an allergic problem. He has nasal allergy, allergic rhinitis, and sinusitis usually with or without infection. The child with a chronic cough or clearing of the throat, sniffling, bloody nose, the allergic, congestive circles under the eyes, etc., are all indicators of the child who has a chronic post-nasal drip with the evidence of some cough coming from the bronchial membranes. And so the immune system is very important to our function.

The elements of the immune or allergic system are antigens and antibodies: Antigens, as I have already mentioned are particles within the air, protein particles which gain entrance to our bodies. Our body is a fortress and it tries to ward off any attempt of bacteria, viruses, thorns, or pollens to grow into our bodies. When these fine substances, called antigens enter the body a reaction occurs. If this happens to be a virus, like measles, that gains entrance to our bodies and breeches our defenses, then the immune system turns on and begins to form antibodies to that substance in order to eradicate it. After a week or two antibodies become available and we test the antibody level to find out the immunity of an individual to measles. As he gets the disease measles, the antibody titer rises and then that gives him immunity to that disease. He doesn't get measles again, by and large, unless he has some defect in his immune production; if he does, he may get measles again or chickenpox or mumps.

These are protective antibodies. There are other forms of antibodies that kind of get fooled and go about the business of not eradicating the foreign organism, but may turn on other tissues in the body and so we can have a destructive effect of antibodies upon tissues we should preserve intact. Also we will have more to say about that.

The blood cells in this immune system are the previously mentioned eosinophils, the basophils which contain bluish staining granules, and the tissue cells, called the mast cells. At the present time our understanding indicates that the mast cells are the ones which bear the brunt of the allergic reaction and their granules contain large amounts of chemical mediators which is primarily histamine among other ones. Mast cells undergoing an allergic reaction de-granulate; they release their chemicals, histamine and others. The histamine makes the blood vessels dilate and the mucous goes out and makes you miserable. It can make you wheeze and go into shock, etc. You've heard of anti-histamine, and so you see how this comes in here.

We've referred to the lymph organs: the tonsils and adenoids. The spleen is a blood forming lymphoid organ. The thymus is a well-known lymphoid organ which previously had been thought to have no function, but we now know has a very vital function in producing the immune cells. The gut is a lymphoid organ, also. Its many feet of meandering lymph tissues provide a large quantity of lymphoid reactive surface, and the appendix, of course, being a part of the gut.

The lymph nodes are those things which swell in kid's necks, and under their jaws, when they have infections or when they have allergies. If you see a child with swollen glands, or the mother points them out, it may be due to some kind of irritation such as allergy in his mucous membranes of the nose and face, or low-grade infection, or some other disorder.

The lymphocytes are single nuclei blood cells which are produced by the immune system and are probably the keys in the building blocks of the whole immune system. There are two forms of theses mall lymphocytes circulating in the blood: the "T" cells and the "B" cells. The "T" cells are so named because they come from the thymus. The "B" cells go to the bursa in the gut. Beta adrenergic receptors are chemical sites in cells which are sensitive to certain chemicals. They apparently have a great deal to do with the allergic reactions.

And so, the immune system that we have is comprised of the lymph nodes, the lymphocytes, the mast cells, etc., and it has the following functions: The first is to defend the body against foreign invaders. If this is active, we have resistance to infection. We don't get measles again; we don't get chickenpox again. Of course, medicine gives lots of immunizations to kids for diphtheria, whooping cough, tetanus, measles, etc., which evokes a reaction of the host and we get resistance to disease. If this system is under-active due to inborn problems of metabolism in which this system does not work, and they fail to produce gamma globulin, which is an antibody which prevents the foreign bacteria and viruses from coming in. When you have a low gamma globulin state in the blood you can get one infection after another, and you have recurrent bacterial infections. Often these children have meningitis 4-5 times, bloodstream infections, recurrent pneumonias, sinusitis, etc., and we administer gamma globulin to these children and help to preserve their lives and for the rest of their lives they have to take it.

If this defense system is overactive, in a simplified way we can think of this as an allergic state, it's turned on excessively and overreacting. This seems to be a very common problem in our society. The child in bio-social decline, the child with a visual problem, the child with minimal brain dysfunction, seems to develop this nonspecific decline in his ability to regulate his immune system. The other function of homeostasis is removal of the old cells within the body; old blood cells, damaged cells, etc., are removed or cleaned up. I had the opportunity of listening to our blood vessels last night over at Dave Dunning's house through an ultra-sound stethoscope. It sounded like Niagara Falls. If you've ever listened to the activity, the noise within your body, you'll find there is a great deal of trauma going on within yourself everyday. You can understand how cells get damaged in their transits and grow old and need to be cleaned out of the system and this is done by this immune system by recognizing a cell that becomes sufficiently damaged or so strange that it is recognized as being foreign to the system.

Over-activity of this system does occur in allergy, and we get an internal allergy to ourselves. We call this auto-immune disease. It's when you are eating yourself up with your allergic system and you may be destroying your own red cells, for instance, and you become anemic due to autoimmune hemolytic anemia. These are very real, definite, pathologic entities. It's to show you the broad scope of the immune or allergic problems.

The surveillance function is vital and certain mutant cells that are produced by radiation and perhaps chemicals within the system of replicating the cells.These mutants are removed by the normally functioning surveillance system in the immune system. Of course when this fails, when a mutant cell fails to be recognized and disposed, then we develop a malignancy. I'll show you a little bit more about the picture in malignancy in a moment, *but there is an immune or allergic aspect to cancer.*

The bone marrow cells start in the bone marrow and they develop into two general forms of white blood cells; lymphocytes or granulocytes. The granulocytes become the cleaner uppers of the system. They engulf bacteria and foreign particle and they form pus. The polymorphous cells and the eosinophils also engulf foreign particles and release their lysosomes which then destroy these foreign protein particles by enzymatic action. And so we have a very important part of the defense mechanism, the phagocytosis. If these cells are not active and if they do not have well-formed membranes that can reach out into pseudopods and make phagosomes then we have a defective resistance due to defective phagocytosis.

The lymphocytes are the drones of the immune system and they form the "T" and "B" cells. The tonsils go about the business of cleaning up the dead killer cells. The "B" cells have as their primary function the formation of antibodies, which look in on the foreign substances and prepare them for phagocytosis. And so the systems work together.

These antibodies are produced by "B" cells, "B"-type lymphocytes. The two main ones to consider are the IgG, the gamma globulin, which provides the resistance to diseases, and the IgE, which is implicated in allergic reactions. This is called skin sensitizing, antibody or reagin. Another, the IgA is interesting because it's a secretory type of antibody and when this is deficient, we have problems within the gut and it is felt that within the first 6-9 months of life the young infant is intolerant of various foods. This is a definite clinical observation. You see lots of food allergy or intolerances in young infants of less than 8-9 months of age. Very often the antigenic load, the allergic load to the child, can be overwhelming if the child is eating great amounts of solid foods, egg protein, etc. early in life before his gut has had a chance to build up a protective layer of IgA antibody. The experience of the child in the first year of life, in regard to antigenic loading, 'can determine how his lymphatic system may react thereafter. You see them in your office with the history of colds, infections and allergies.

Let us look at the allergic reaction. This is apparently what happens. We use the term "allergy" but often we don't know what we're saying. What does it mean? The mast cell in the tissues becomes sensitized by prior exposure to something. If it's egg protein, for instance, the egg protein may sensitize the mast cell so that on re-exposure to the egg protein it will then fire off. This prior exposure is very important. If you're 30 years of age, how and when your system fires off depends, to a large extent, on what happened to you during your entire previous 30 years of life with regard to the antigenic exposure that one's had. For instance, if you've never been around ragweed, you'll not be allergic to ragweed, but after you've been in ragweed country for a year or two, then you can become allergic to rag weed. And so this sensitized mast cell reacts with the IgE, which is a physio-allergic type of antibody and the antigen which may be egg white protein, ragweed, dust, or whatever to evoke the release of histamine from these granules in this mast cell. Then the histamine does something to the cell membrane, causing the cell membrane to lose its electric potential and it depolarizes, and you get damage to the cells. When you have damage to the cell, blood vessels dilate, mucous forms, and all sorts of things happen; smooth muscles contract, etc. So there is the mast cell, and here are the two allergic antibodies, which have been formed by prior exposure, on the wall of the cell, and here is the protein substance which has gained entrance to the body by breathing it, eating it or injecting it and then is the aforementioned reaction occurs.

The allergic reaction, the degranulation of the mastcell, can be turned on by traumatic factors also: cold, exercise or emotional factors can also apparently play in here to cause the release of this whole mechanism. Thus we have some evidence that there is a mixture together, a concept of loading on the individual from his emotional and physical environment as well as from his antigenic, immune environment.

Further characterizing the allergic reaction, this is what is thought to happen. If we are talking about people who usually have a family history of allergy, then we can postulate a diminished ability of their systems, a diminished reactivity of the beta adrenergic system. There is an enzyme in the cell membranes called adenylyl cyclase. This enzyme is the key to kicking off are action involving ATP, which is the energy molecule within the cells. This enzyme, when present and stimulated, kicks off a reaction that lets cyclic AMP (cAMP) be formed, and bolsters the defense of the cell membrane and preserves its integrity, if you will.

Certain other things also happen in the presence of this substance. Sugar is metabolized properly; glycogenolysis. Fat is metabolized properly; lypolysis. Smooth muscle relaxes, and does not go into spasm. And so you begin to see the implication: perhaps in the smooth muscles of the eye, smooth muscle in the bronchial walls, states of obesity—underfat or overfat—and states of disordered carbohydrate metabolism related to the immune or allergic process. If working properly, then the cAMP does all of these things and causes these things to occur. Here we have an antagonistic effect with histamine. Histamine trying to break down this cell membrane, the internal workings of cAMP bolstering the cell wall and so you can see the concept of relative balance here just as we have in the whole body. What the eventual result will be with that child may be determined by hereditary factors regarding the mechanism of this bio-chemistry here, the antigenic loading, prior exposure, etc. here releasing histamine, and the state of the child's physiology as of the moment.

The catecholamines are adrenaline, and ephedrine. These are the neuro-mediators: norepinephrine, epinephrine. They activate this system. If a child's diet is not sufficient, if he has some disease and perhaps he's not getting enough protein in his diet, then he may have an acidotic tendency, which blockades this system. Antitoxin from bacteria blockades this system, also. So we see nutritional aspects, disease aspects, and infectious, allergic and hereditary aspects. This is very rough and crude, but it's designed to, hopefully, give you an appreciation for the multiplicity of factors that interact to determine what happens to the integrity of cell membranes and the chemical mediators involved.

Going back to this concept of the child who is in bio-social decline, things just aren't going his way; he can't hack it; things get worse;

he develops allergies if he didn't have them; he develops infections if he didn't have them; the family-child relationships are suffering; he's developing visual problems along the way if he didn't have them. He's caught in this cycle of being unable to achieve, unable to feel right, having one problem after another: activity, visual, social relationship problems, etc.

This may be what happens in some of these children with bio-social decline. We get a cyclic piling up sort of effect. Stress of one sort or another, be it visual, nutritional, emotional, infectious, physical: producing a failure to cope which then seems to be related to the total load mechanisms of goal setting and goal satisfaction. Lowering the norepinephrine, the catecholamines within the brain, result in a clinical state of depression in activation, and the reticular activating system declines. A failure to cope because of this: non-motivation, non-trying, insufficient attention to task, inability to follow through and producing more failure to cope and lowered brain norepinephrine, fewer catecholamines, the production of allergies and the now unbalanced histamine which goes ahead and causes the dissolution of membrane integrity, the production of allergies, the lowered resistance of the membranes, the infections coming and sometimes then the failure of the fat and carbohydrate system to work right producing obesity in some, hypoglycemia in others, asthma in some, etc. There are lots of open spots in this system and this is not gospel, but this as a proposed mechanism that fits with the clinical observations so far.

In the matter of cancer, it may have a great deal to do with what we eat. When we ate eggs, wheat, citrus, and milk as a baby. What our heredity was. What antigenic loading we've had over the years. How our immune system has been programmed to take care of foreign invaders and mutants within the system. In cancer a tumor mass grows and produces protein particles which are flooding the system. These protein antigens form a cancer in the spleen and lymph nodes and produce an antibody response, the "B" and the "T" cells, and produce the lymphocytes. The "B" cells produce antibodies against the tumor antigen. These combine and the "T" cells, which ordinarily would kill these foreign cells in the body, should go ahead as killer cells and take care of this tumor. But for some reason there is so much flooding of the body with this antigen that it seems to block the effect of these cells, and the tumor goes on its merry way. The individual is a victim of a hyper state of allergy or immunity here, but it cannot be affected and it is blocked. Therefore in some cases of tumors, removing the primary tumor mass is very helpful because it reduces the vast bulk of this antigen and allows this immune mechanism to be effective. There is no doubt that there are other factors in here we don't understand as yet but you can see the close approximation of "allergy" with some of the basic problems of mankind.

Recently there was some play about the use of the bacille Calmette-Guérin (BCG) vaccination in the press activating the immune system so that it would take care of cancers. This, of course, is preliminary yet; we don't know how it's going to come out. But that type of thing is what's involved in the understanding of the whole mechanism of resistance and susceptibility, not only to the effects of a bad teacher but to the effects of pollen or the effects of a tumor within the body.

The host is subject to a large antigenic load throughout its life. It's coming through the nose, as dust particles, pollen and other elements in the environment. It's continually being swallowed into the gut. These antigens are being eaten. The degree and duration of antigenic exposure has a great deal to do with how our immune system works; whether it fires off inadequately or in an abnormal fashion. The less antigen exposure, the less antigen load, the better the child functions in general, and the more his immune system develops. And so we try to prevent allergy, if you will, from the very moment of conception or even before. We tell people with a strong family history of allergy to avoid ingesting large amounts of the known allergic foods during pregnancy. We perhaps try to have them avoid strong dust and pollen in the environments during that time. This is a vital factor.

The neurological function of the individual is important in the host in determining his resistance or susceptibility to the immune dysfunction, the emotional factors, the effect of nutrition and the visual factors. I have seen children in my practice who have lost their allergies completely under vision therapy. I have seen children in my practice whose allergies have been markedly diminished when they began wearing plus lenses. I have seen children in my practice who developed allergies under vision training, who developed chronic, allergic tension fatigue states and who were then treated from the allergic standpoint with either a food manipulation, antihistamine therapy or injection therapy, and then they were able to go on and tolerate vision therapy in office with excellent results in a very short period of time, and so these are the inter-relationships of your profession and mine.

The children who have non-evident allergy—the symptoms are not gross enough to be found by anyone—very often develop evident allergy at a later date in their lives. We must think of children from the whole-life span. What kind of adults are they going to become? What kind of job holders? What kind of parents for their own children?

These are some of the ways we have of treating allergy. The first one on the list is antibiotics. That seems odd but it stresses again the common coexistence of infections in the respiratory mucous membrane with the underlying allergic disorder. We see time and again that the child who has an infection must have the infection cleared and then the allergic underlying disorder should be taken care of, and so antibiotics are a very important part of the therapy. They can be abused, of course, but there are some children that we just can't get well without the use of these.

The antihistamine drugs are an over-the-counter item in very weak forms. I think these are drugs that should not be used when other methods of therapy are available and effective, but there are some individuals who are highly sensitive to certain antihistamines and it's necessary to use them in order to clear them up. It's very wise to use them on a temporary basis to gain a foothold on the problem. The catecholamines are adrenaline, ephedrine and norepinephrine. There are some people who take Sudafed, or something like that, and who are only able to function in the classroom when they have this. And so you see that Ritalin isn't the only drug that needs to be used. Incidentally, Ritalin may be in this category. The Methylxanthines are drugs like Aminophylline that are used to treat asthma or bronchial constriction. They work in a slightly different way than the catecholamines but they involve the same system I have shown you,

The cortico-steroids, the cortisone-like drugs, are highly effective and they're like an automobile; they can do an awful lot of damage but that doesn't mean you stop driving. They are very helpful in getting a foothold on some of these problems. There are some children with allergic disorders and learning disorders that I have on cortico-steroids for a year or two in very small doses. Cromolyn is a new agent which is not available in our country at this time but you may be hearing about it and your patients may be taking it within the next year or two. It's called Intal in Englan. It seems to work in asthmatics particularly by stabilizing those mast cells so that the degranulization doesn't take place and the other chemical mediators are not released.

The desensitizing injections are the allergy shots which, again, are an interesting subject of discussion. Sometimes it is necessary to use these to get children well. The allergy injections are protein antigens that the child reacts to on skin testing generally. These are introduced under the skin and build up the IgG antibodies, so-called blocking antibodies which block the effect of the IgE, or the reagin antibodies. These injections can produce all of the symptoms that you're trying to prevent. For instance, I had a child with nosebleeds. He had nosebleeds everyday of his life. We gave him a single injection of an allergy solution containing the substances to which he reacted; and he had no more nosebleeds. We kept giving him the injections, and then about 6 months later he began to have nosebleeds again. We had passed his tolerance limit and so we had to back off at that point, and when we did, his nosebleeds went away. This happens very frequently.

Naturally avoidance is a primary way of reducing the load on the child. Very often I see children with visual problems who are receiving vision therapy and who accelerate their response to vision therapy when we have them avoid the substances to which they are reacting and which is causing them to have a load. And so you see, we have a mutual way of helping the patient here.

The use of megavitamins in some patients seems to turn off the allergic process also as does taking care of family problems, counseling, etc. Perceptual motor therapy sometimes is helpful also. I have mentioned the children who respond to lenses.

I would like to just then leave you with an impression that this matter of allergy is nota vague substance, a vague thing that you may have heard about or had once in a while in your own life, but it's a very real entity. Immunology is a science which is rapidly uncovering the mechanisms of action and explaining why all the things we've been doing through the years in medicine are helpful or not helpful. It involves a consideration of the most basic factors of life involving cellular metabolism and cellular resistance to cancer. Most importantly of all, an appreciation and an understanding of allergy and its follow up infection can help you to do a better job, in caring for the little children with the snotty noses in your office.

Inter-professional Relationships

Dr. Greenstein has taken a leadership role in trying to bring together our professions. This is a monumental chore and I'd like to see it approached on a national level in both our professions. One thing that he did was to stimulate me to write some questions to be asked by the parent or the professional about the child's particular pediatrician or family physician. I thought that some of these questions might be of interest to you, therefore I thought I'd read them to you. If you ask these of a physician, they might be of help in discovering whether that physician has experience and knowledge with children and with the kind of problems you're working with.

The first question is based upon the fact that some information about the child's mental sphere status quo is important. The first question to a physician: ***Do you order and obtain psychological testing on children?*** The next question pertains to his examination of the child: ***Do you conduct or obtain a developmentally oriented pediatric-neurological examination***? There is a world of difference between the adult-oriented neurological exam and the developmental pediatric neurological exam. As I haves aid, I view a lot of our work as overlapping in this neurological sphere.

The third question might be something like this: ***Do you prescribe the following when indicated: anti-convulsive medications, stimulants, tranquilizers, nutritional therapy and megavitamins?*** This gives a physician a clear choice in making yes or no answers , and by assessing the answers, you'll know something about whether you wish this particular child to attend that physician or not.

Another question might be: ***Will you see this child at least as often as every few months to supervise his treatment?*** Because the child who is placed on Phenobarbitol and sent away and seen a year later is obviously in the same position as giving him a lens which may need to be changed more often than every year.

The last question I have modeled after some of your vision optometric questions: ***Will my child's teacher receive a report from you that she can understand?*** These questions, I think, may help in making physicians aware that you are aware of the importance of those areas.

I had wanted to discuss vitamins and nutrition during this hour, but I would also like to field some questions from the audience, if you have them, to see if there are any areas that you have that you'd like to have me discuss. Is there anything that you have on your minds that you'd like to bring up at this point that I might be able to answer?

MEMBER: Can we get better care of the patient regarding his complaints by going directly to a specialist rather than to a general physician? It seems like they go to the GP but it stops at that point and I'm in a bad position to say, "He advised you incorrectly." I can't do that.

DR. WUNDERLICH: I think you have to -- there are certain things where you have to take a stand. I think you should go first to the family physician. Then if there is still a continuing problem that you are aware of, then I think you owe it to those people to suggest another opinion. Another opinion is always O.K. That's why we have the American system of medicine.

MEMBER: All right, now if that's the case, let's say that in the case of sinus pain around the eye, should it be an ENT source, an allergist source, or a pediatric source?

DR. WUNDERLICH: That will differ in your community. You have to know your people and what their biases are in their practice. One way to do this has been to say: The last two patients that I've had with these complaints have seen these physicians—one, two, three, and they've had good results. Perhaps you may wish to do this.

MEMBER: I guess what I'm trying to get at is—with these sub-specialties, would their particular philosophical approach differ sufficiently so that I would have more success if I steered the patient to one direction or another?

DR. WUNDERLICH: I would suspect that most of the time the ear, nose and throat doctors are rather anatomically oriented and the allergists are more apt to be functionally oriented, although many of them stop, too, at just an awareness of asthma, hay fever, and eczema. However, the newer allergy meetings are incorporating much of the data which I gave you today.

MEMBER: How about the pediatrician in this case?

DR. WUNDERLICH: The pediatrician is apt to do allergy. There are many pediatricians who do allergy and many pediatricians who are excellent ear, nose and throat practitioners. The problem of middle ear fluid, I haven't brought it up today, but this is extremely important. It seems to depress the whole function of the brain and the visual system whenever we have a lingering, middle ear effusion. These may require placement of mechanical drainage tubes or selected adenoidectomies at times. Usually, as I said this morning, the surgical problems can be saved to the last. With the use of high vitamin dosages: antibiotics, antihistamines, etc., we can usually manage these without resorting to surgery. Let me just say, in regard to these vitamin dosages, we can get into as much detail on this as you would like to. Let me know what you would like to do.

MEMBER: What about a problem such as chronic blepharitis in an early adolescent when the physician seems to ignore it?

Dr. WUNDERLICH: The child may not be hurting with it and the question is whether there is an appreciation of small deviations from normal or not. You and I know that the small deviation, be it in the visual system or in the health system, can be of great importance. It is a matter that if you feel it may be important, then I think you owe it to that child and your patient to stand up for it and to see to it that they get an opinion about it from another source. If you don't, I think you're a coward.

MEMBER: I would be interested in the amount and distribution of vitamins in the megavitamins.

DR. WUNDERLICH: Some of your colleagues here very nicely went out today and took care of that. It's right here in this bottle. It says, "To be taken in case of allergy, chills, etc." and so if you're weak in the knees, you can get some of these little sugar pellets here they call megavitamins. But actually the megavitamins consist of the harmless B and C vitamins. These start with B-1, we often use large amounts of that, B-2 somewhat. B-6 is one of the key ones, Pyridoxine. We use anywhere from 100 mg to 400 mg per day of vitamin B-6, Pyridoxine, and we haven't seen any side effects from its administration. B-6 is a vitamin that is working in many of the metabolic pathways and is involved in most of the vitamin-dependent disorders. This vitamin was missing from SMA milk infant formulae in the early days of formula. The children drinking formula had convulsions associated with the lack of B-6 in the formula, and so you can see what a profound metabolic agent it is. That's B-6.

Vitamin C has a long history and you're all aware of the controversy regarding it with the scientific community and Linus Pauling. Suffice it to say, much of the effect of Vitamin C appears to be on this immunologic problem, the allergic problem, rather than upon the common cold. The question comes down to—what is a common cold? It's very difficult to find what a common cold is anymore because most of the colds appear to be allergy related and I use the word cold in quotation marks. At any rate, we see children whose lymph tissue melts away under the administration of large amounts of vitamin C. We see children who cease having their "colds" and/or allergy once they take this optimal amount of Vitamin C. You have to find this optimal amount for yourself. For each individual it seems to vary. We have children who lose their allergies and infections when they take 125-250 mg of Vitamin C, once, twice or thrice a day. We have others who require 1,000 mg 3 times a day. This is about as high as I've gone in the pediatric age group.

We do see some toxic effects from Vitamin C, although it's rare. These can be diarrhea, anal irritation, urinary frequency, skin rash resembling prickly heat. Interestingly enough down in the Old South where we see Florida prickly heat quite frequently, and anywhere in the tropics, Vitamin C is an old remedy for this and has been used for many years.

Another main agent is Niacinamide, which is used in the megavitamin package at this time. It is a package at this time and one has to juggle it about and find what the best ratio of elements is for the individual. The Niacinamide is used in doses of 12 grams, 3 times a day, for a child of 3-5 years up to perhaps 20 grams of Niacin a day which is a massive, massive dose in older people. To some extent, one can take an individual and perform a test like the Hoffer-Osmund Test[4] and titrate his results with Niacin therapy. This test measures perceptual distortions, depression and other mental aberrations. It's really a remarkable substance. It has a calming action, too, for the hyperactive child. We use the Niacinamide usually in children rather than Niacin because of the severe flushing effect that one gets with the Niacin. Someone showed me a very severe flushing effect very recently and if you've ever had it from Niacin it's like one of these flushes that women get when they haven't any menstrual period anymore—only worse.

The other agent that is commonly used is Pantothenic Acid or Calcium Pantothenate. This is used in doses of perhaps 100-400 mg per day. This agent, in my experience, is the least useful of all these elements. In the experience of Allan Cott from New York, it's quite helpful. Again, the most frequent side effect that I see here is an increase in the hyper activity of the child. However, one must be careful. If one does not get a proper dosage, he may not get the proper effect. When I first started using Calcium Pantothenate, or Niacinamide, I was creeping up on the dosage, basically being a conservative person, and I was finding I was not getting the effects. When I went to the full dosage, I began to get the effects and often we will get an effect after a month or two, possibly earlier, with the megavitamin treatment, and then reach a plateau. At the time of that plateauing—let's say when hyperactivity is decreasing or attention span is improving and the behavior is becoming lovable, then one needs to either change the dose at the time of the plateau, or invoke some other therapeutic intervention.

Then we use other agents in combination. We use minerals of various kinds. We investigate the hair and do a hair analysis from the nape of the neck. The most common finding we find is a lack of sodium <u>and potassium</u> in the hair. Sometimes we see deficient calcium,

---

4. *This test is a psychiatric test that was used in the 70's but seems to have fallen out of favor at the time of this publication, 2010.*

magnesium, manganese or zinc and then we treat that accordingly. The hair analysis gives us a picture of the child over some length of time whereas a blood test would just give us the immediate finding of the moment. The hair analysis also allows us to know about the state of cadmium, chromium, lead, and mercury in the hair. These are the more toxic minerals.

MEMBER: Does the flushing that comes with Niacine have any relationship to the need for the agent?

DR. WUNDERLICH: Apparently not, because you see it very, very frequently and often as you give it, it tends to go awayand yet if you drop the dose at all the symptoms return. It's a direct effect of the agent. As a matter of fact, it's used as a vasodilator in some cerebral spastic states and in peripheral arterial disease.

MEMBER: Does our present culture have more allergy than in the past?

DR. WUNDERLICH: I don't know of any good studies that can answer it scientifically. It appears to me that in just in my brief span of pediatric practice of some 11 years that I'm seeing many more allergic problems now than I did then. One always wonders about the increased ability to recognize it, of course, and so I don't have the answer for you. I think, however, that the environmental pollutants in the air, the particles I have referred to, are making more irritable tissues and perhaps making the allergies, which were more latent before, more apparent. There is no question that the diet of the society is going to the dogs and at the present time the American public feeds its dogs much better than it feeds itself; for the first time in history.

MEMBER: How long do you employ the megavitamins?

DR. WUNDERLICH: The duration of treatment with megavitamin therapy is, the longer the better. Once you hit the effective regimen, then you maintain it for an indefinite time; the longer the better. You will see results within 1-6 months. A trial therapy should be over at least several months before one says that it's not effective. As yet, we've not had enough information to know what sub fractions of children with problems are the best candidates for this. It appears, however, that those who are withdrawn, who tend to withdraw from the stresses of life, who are introverted and live within themselves and who are more paranoid are the better candidates for response from the treatment.

I started to mention that these diseases of civilization that we were discussing would be of interest to you. The primitive tribes in Africa are remarkably free from what we call the diseases of civilization. These are arteriosclerosis, stomach ulcers, duodenal ulcers, diverticulitis of the colon, polyps of the colon—polyps are a large problem in civilized society—cancer of the colon, gall bladder disease, diabetes mellitus, sugar diabetes and myopia. Whether allergies are in this or not, I'm not sure. Mostly we have evidence on these gastro-intestinal diseases; I suspect it is. As the primitive natives grow closer to civilized areas and adopt their dietary habits these diseases begin to show up in a direct line ratio to the amount of time the natives spend in civilized areas. And so it appears that these, indeed, are diseases of civilization and, as such, have perhaps some common denominator with the myopia problem in which you are dealing.

MEMBER: What about Vitamin E?

DR. WUNDERLICH: Vitamin E, I didn't mention. Perhaps that's because I'm somewhat biased against it. I use it. It is used in the megavitamin package. However it's not one of the main agents and my personal feeling is that it's not often helpful. I've not seen any harm from it as yet except in high doses where it appears to make the individual somewhat sluggish and perhaps to have a lowering of the blood pressure effect. The dosages I commonly use are 100 units perhaps 2-3 times a day; usually not over that unless we're dealing with an adult.

MEMBER: What about Vitamin B-12?

DR. WUNDERLICH: Vitamin B-12 plays a minor part but a definite part and can be used with certain individuals. As you know, B-12 has an effect on some individuals. From the strictly scientific standpoint, B-12 should be used for the treatment of pernicious anemia and nothing else. However, I think the full story is not known on that yet. I think that B-12 does have a definite effect on some individuals, the optimal amounts are not known. More important is Vitamin B-15, which is pandemic acid which is of great importance and which is not available in this country. This appears to have a strong anti-asthma effect and a strong effect in normalizing hyperactivity and increasing oxygen and the flow to the tissues and in bringing out the deficient language development, speech development, of the child.

MEMBER: Are the megavitamins getting to the cause of these problems?

DR. WUNDERLICH: It appears they are. Traditional medicine has to do with problems that hurt and that prevent you from going about your business, problems that are severe enough to make you go to the doctor. On the other hand, there are people who are walking around and are going to develop problems in the future. They are the ones, perhaps, who are trying to use their eyes and minds to the best advantage in the classroom but who have incipient or low-grade illness. The question is how can we reach the point of optimal health for all of us? One of the things that has happened in the nutritional aspects of our society over the past 70 years is that there has been a marked drop in the ingestion of starches, complex carbohydrates and a marked increase in the consumption of simple sugars. As a matter of fact, it's very difficult to get away from eating simple sugar in your diet. If you'll look on your box of salt you'll find that one of the ingredients of the salt package is sugar.

As that happens and as these simple sugars are eaten, sugar and vitamins and minerals are combined in nature, and so as you get a high incidence of these simple sugars which are stripped of their values, you do get these deficiencies. And at the same time because they provide calories, you do automatically have a lowered protein diet and a lowered vitamin and mineral intake. Over the months and years, apparently this has some effect.

Here are some curves to show you the result of eating various food substances, all of which areisoglucogenic quantities, that is, they are capable of releasing equivalent amounts of calories. On the top you see simple sugar, glucose. You see the marked rise in the blood sugar which occurs, and the fall off. This is the important thing; the more rapid the blood sugar rises, the more rapid it changes, the more stress it is upon the endocrine system of the body. And so, every time you ingest a molecule of sugar you are having this rapid stress, this rapidly absorbed substance which is like accelerating 60 miles per hour in your car within a few seconds. Bread, which is a more complex carbohydrate, produces a lower rise a little later. The apple, which is an apple-fruit sugar, gives you a lesser rise. The ingestion of protein gives you a minor rise but a nice, sustained, long production of blood glucose. This is the key, then, to the treatment of children with these problems of high protein diets to smooth these out so you don't have these valleys, these great valleys and mountains stressing their metabolic machinery, the endocrine system.

There is an antagonistic role here between the pancreas and the adrenal cortex as we begin to look closely into the system. Of course, the cortical hormones are hydrocortisone and the pancreatic secretion is insulin. These tend to be more or less balancing agents, one for the other, within the body. When one is released, then the other has to be released to have a dampening effect. And so there enters a complex system of endocrine changes involving the autonomic nervous system also just from the simple matter of ingesting a little bit of sugar. Now what can happen with this delicate balance? You can start with the ingestion of sugar. It's absorbed from the gut very quickly, the simple sugars, protein more slowly. Glucose goes to the liver unchanged and passes out into the blood, and there is a rise in the blood sugar. The pancreas reacts to this, the Islets of Langerhans, secreting Insulin, and so we have glucose and insulin going to the liver, back to the liver in the portal vein. The glucose, in the presence of insulin, forms animal starch, or glycogen, which is a storehouse for us. And so the liver piles up with glycogen which is a way of storing the sugar as starch. The result of this is that a similar amount of glucose comes out of the liver and the glucose then goes to the tissues and it's metabolized in what is known as glycolysis. As it is used by the brain and the body, the glucose lowers and you have lowered blood glucose. The adrenal cortex senses this, through the pituitary system incidentally, senses this, probably actually in the hypo-thalamus, and releases the hydrocortisone which then acts in the liver to break down the glycogen already made there to produce more sugar. And so you can see everything that goes on set in motion by the simple act of ingesting the sugar.

Now at a more minute level here is some of the bio-chemistry involved and the cellular metabolism of every cell in the body. This will be the retina, the brain, the cells of the little toe, the pancreas, the adrenal cortex, etc. And so if you have an imbalanced state, a state of chronic, cellular malnutrition, that goes on and you have these cells working sub-optimally, and months and years go along, and you have sub-optimal performance. We have glucose again coming in and being stored for when it's needed, being metabolized in the cells to pyruvate end products here. Here protein can come in and contribute to this blood glucose. And so if we eat protein, then we get it this way in a slow dribble. We get it another way and then we get it in peaks and valleys. Fat also can be burned, but must be burned when this is active. This system must be active for this to be active.

We get two sources of two carbon fragments which are further metabolized in the all-important tri-carboxylic acid cycle, or Krebs cycle, and here is where the energy comes out of this business. If this is blocked we would not have the production of energy; for instance if we have no Vitamin B-1. Enzymes involving these B vitamins and the minerals: magnesium and others are instrumental in nearly every stop of this, and so you see how the megavitamin therapy applies to the actual cellular metabolism here.

Here's an example[5] of some blood sugar curves that we see. The one on the top might be normal. It rises, reaches a peak within a half hour to an hour and then comes down and levels out. For this individual, the peak has dipped too low, indicating that perhaps there has been too much insulin fired at this point. The insulin is released by the rapidity of the rise. The change in the blood level is what triggers this rather than the absolute level. Too much has been secreted; it's been a little bit off, like the eyes being a little off focus, and you have the hypoglycemic phase here. Here you have an erratic sort of curve. Remember all the things that are happening with insulin release and the hydrocortisone release and all the other factors necessary for that to happen. This leads into a very markedly abnormal one in which you have, perhaps, a little insulin here, maybe a little more here and an erratic, kind of a chugging motor going along. There are cases where the sugar may not have been actually absorbed at all. And then there are the typical hypoglycemic curves in which you have the hair trigger pancreas, a pancreas which has so often been insulted and caused to fire by the daily ingestion of carbohydrates, simple carbohydrates, that it becomes trigger happy and fires too fast, too much and gets the individual into hyperinsu-

---

5. *Editor's note: we do not have access to the original slides shown by the author but felt the text was valuable to keep as is.*

linism and low blood sugar hypoglycemia. And the final curve is the diabetic curve which very often follows the state of hypoglycemia. Very often if we look retrospectively back into diabetics' histories we find that they have had hypoglycemia preceding the development of their diabetes. In other words, that the system has been taxed so much, it fires off and it becomes a trigger happy pancreatic mechanism and then finally gives out and is unable to function, and so you have no way to metabolize sugar in the body and you have all the complication of sugar diabetes. Are there any questions?

MEMBER: Are these the results of the fasting glucose tests?

DR. WUNDERLICH: The fasting glucose test would be where you start. First the patient is given a sugar load, it rises and then follows whichever curve it may do. Is that clear?

MEMBER: If you had a fasting glucose test, would it show on the chart?

DR. WUNDERLICH: No. These are only the results of loading of the patient with a glucose load. The fasting tests—these are absolutely essential to a diagnosis of the problem. The fasting glucose test may or may not help you. That is, taking it in the morning after an overnight fast. The values of fasting blood tests may be completely normal and you may still have these problems. As a matter of fact, your glucose tolerance curve—5-hour or 6-hour—may be normal and you may still have the problem. Sometimes we have to resort to what we call the stress-activated glucose tolerance test. Here again, you see a similarity with vision. You may not see the vision problem until you subject that child to some more visual stress—and then something comes up. We can take a child with a perfectly compatible history but he's distractible, his symptoms are intermittent, on and off. He has a positive family history of diabetes. He craves and eats sweets all the time and craves sweets and water. You check him on the glucose tolerance test and it's normal, but he still has the symptoms. He even grows faint in the afternoon, perhaps at 4PM or does poorly in the late morning. Then you repeat the test after stressing him by activity. You can have him run up and down, jog up and down in place for 5 minutes. And then you can have him hyperventilate. Or you can subject him to cold.

Or you can give him some kind of psychic stress. You will then see the development of hypoglycemia.

MEMBER: Do you care to comment upon the relationship between low blood sugar and allergies?

DR. WUNDERLICH: Yes, there is a definite association between the two. There are papers that have been published on this. Low blood sugar is more common in allergic patients and vice versa. However, there are some individuals in whom they are completely separate, and so you have overlapping populations. If you try to take the posture that these allergic individuals are hyperinsulinisms, it just doesn't work out all the time. There are some allergic individuals who have nothing to do with low blood sugar. On the other hand, it's very interesting.

All of the medications we use for asthmatics, for instance, elevate the blood sugar: Adrenalin, Ephedrine, Xanthine drugs, etc. Of course, the answer probably is that it's tied up with adenyl cyclase system, the enzyme system in the cell, getting this system going and then it has different effects. Remember I spoke about the sugar metabolism there and on the bronchial vessels. There may be a stronger effect in one direction than in another with some individuals, perhaps hereditary patterns or prior experiences in their lives.

These then are the culprits that we see. They all start with the letter "C". It's civilization, carbohydrates and it's cane sugar. The cola-holics, the cereal-holics and the alcoholics and the caffeine-holics and all of this type. All of those are what we find in what we call the American corner-kid syndrome, some of which have hypoglycemia and others who do not have perhaps the hereditary pattern and do not get into hypoglycemia but may develop other problem areas.

These are some of the causes that we see carbohydrate related, mentioned the catarrh or the allergy or infections. The confusion some of these children show after they ingest these things, some may actually cause convulsions from low blood sugar, states of disorientation, episodic crying, disinhibition and the craving of sweets. The craving is amazing that many of these children have; they just have to have them. Of course, what they're doing is they are repetitively stimulating their system, getting highs and lows and filling in the gaps by raiding the corner candy box.

Interestingly enough, most of the cold drinks have caffeine in them and caffeine acts as a stimulant here and you end up with the same effect as if you'd eaten sugar. And so most of the time these children are getting the sugar and the caffeine. The caffeine is present in candy bars, in the Hershey Bars, for instance, both regular and bittersweet, and present in other items.

Dr. Philip H. Taylor
Nutrition and Vision
1979

Lecture I

Ladies and gentlemen, my discussion is basically going to be in three parts: I'm going to talk about 1) vision as related to nutrition, 2) some salient points of nutrition in general, and 3) learning disabilities related to nutrition and the treatment thereof.

When I'm through today you'll have to ask yourself: Do I live in a healthy house? A healthy house has walls made out of oatmeal, the roof was whole wheat crackers, the chimney is real bottles of milk, the pathway leading up to the health house has carrots, turnips and other vegetables which boys and girls who want to grow big and strong can hardly get along without. And then look at this unhealthy house. The wallpaper is out of hotcakes, doorsteps out of hot biscuits, and soda pop chimneys.

We're going to talk about the eye and vision, and although most of you know the anatomy of the eye, I'm going to talk about some features that should be reiterated. First let's look at the capillaries in the eye. We know the capillaries carry the blood and oxygen to the eye. But it's important to know the capillaries have a negative charge and the cells passing through those capillaries also have a negative charge. As the red cells and the other cells are passing single file through those very fine capillaries, they need a little more propulsion than the propulsive effect of the heart so the negativity of the capillary wall and the cell give that propulsive capability, just like putting two like ends of a magnet together and trying to hold them together. The capillaries are 99% of all the blood vessels in the body so you've got to keep the red cells marching single file through those capillaries.

Dr. Raeford, an Atlanta ophthalmologist, can't stress the importance of capillaries enough in his treatment. He has found by taking actual photographs of the retina that sometimes the simple expedient of putting a patient on a good nutritional diet improves the passage of the red cells through those capillaries. If one is not paying attention to good nutrition and one is getting short on supplements, the capillary wall begins to become neutral or even positively charged, and if the cells are negative then there is attraction, and not only are the cells attracted to the capillary walls but also minerals such as calcium. You begin to see perhaps how arteriosclerosis begins to build up.

The choroid contains more zinc than any other part of the body in concentration and in that layer of the choroid is collagen. Collagen is made up of four amino acids and the amino acids are also bound together by co-factors: magnesium, manganese, copper, and Vitamin E. You have to get these things in your diet in adequate amounts to maintain the support for these capillaries. You're supposed to get those from good nutritious foods which is becoming more and more difficult to find. Today, hopefully, I'm going to be able to explode this myth that the American diet is adequate because that's just a lot of bunk. It's impossible for anyone to be getting an adequate diet in the U.S. today unless you are growing your entire food intake, and I'm saying all of it. The way foods are grown and processed today, you get a depleted diet.

I will mention some of the vitamins and how important they are. Vitamin B1 is important to the eye because the eye has a very high rate of glucose metabolism because it's an extension of the central nervous system which requires high amounts of glucose; 25% of all available glucose is to operate that little 3-pound piece of machinery. B1 is extremely important in glucose metabolism, and you want glucose metabolism to be moving in its proper way.

Backtracking a little bit, you can understand that the eye has been considered very important through the ages, even before recorded history apparently. Hindus believe the eye is the window of the soul. The Vedas of the Hindus express the belief of the possibility of transmitting good or evil by means of a look–the old evil eye. Even in the bible: the lap of the body is the eye. It follows that if your eye is sound your whole body will be filled with light, but if your eye is diseased your whole body will be all darkness. If the eye is not functioning properly you will have an impairment of learning and educational processing.

B2 has been found to help maintain adequate tear secretion. Other things that seem to help are iodine in adequate amounts. One of your colleagues, Dr. Lane, in a recent report to the Optical Society of America, feels that chromium may be related to the worsening of myopia. He found there was a particular pattern that seemed to correlate with the worsening of myopia, and that the pattern was to see very high calcium on the hair analysis and lowered chromium. Just because you have high calcium on a hair analysis, it does not follow that you have adequate calcium in your body. High calcium on a hair analysis generally means that a great percentage of that calcium is insoluble. If your body needs calcium in a hurry it's not going to get it from that source. You may actually be deficient in calcium. In following these patients, as chromium values go down, his findings are that myopia tends to worsen. The connection between chromium and calcium is not directly known.

One of the most important vitamins in the eye is Vitamin P or bioflavonoids. Bioflavonoids reduce blood cell clumping. Bioflavonoids also protect Vitamin C from destructive elements so you can take less Vitamin C if you take bioflavonoids. Aldose reductase is an enzyme utilized in the body to change glucose to another kind of carbohydrate called sorbitol. You'll see sorbital as an artificial sweetener in gum and other foods. That is a natural biochemical seen in the body. Glucose can be changed to sorbitol. The particular importance to this in the eye is that the aldose reductase may be a factor in cataract formation. Too much aldose reductase in the eye increases the changing of glucose to sorbital, and sorbital is thought to be one of the factors to promote cataracts. This is extremely important to the diabetic because, the diabetic has an incidence of cataracts six times greater than the normal population. It would seem, especially with a diabetic, that bioflavonoids are extremely important. Also important of the eye bioflavonoids is that hemorrhages are reduced, which are usually more frequent in the diabetic. Bioflavonoids strengthen the wall of the capillary and they also decrease the permeability of the capillary wall. I can say from personal experience that the use of bioflavonoids in these conditions can be very dramatic. Patients who have hemorrhages in their eyes are generally very frightened people. They're afraid that if they sneeze or cough or miss the curb on the street they're going to have another hemorrhage. This is something that can not only reduce the hemorrhage but can give them peace of mind when they know this. Bioflavonoids are found in fairly great amounts in the white portion of an orange or citrus fruits.

Off and on through history I notice that Vitamin D and calcium have been linked with the reduction of myopia. Dr. Knapp, who is an ophthalmologist in New York, has been treating myopia with massive dosages of Vitamin D and calcium. He uses about 50,000 units of Vitamin D on a daily basis and he will give it for as long as 6 months before having a little rest period. This is not the story you'll generally hear. Vitamin D, a fat soluble vitamin, is supposed to be feared as a vitamin which will cause problems in too great of dosages. Back in the 1940's they used to treat arthritis using dosages up to 330,000 units of Vitamin D. There are very few cases of Vitamin D toxicity on record. I don't want to sound as if I'm advocating everyone to take large amounts of Vitamin D, but the idea that Vitamin D will cause severe reactions, I believe, is overrated. Dr. Knapp is a very careful kind of researcher who has gone so far as to make castings of the front of the eye in conjunction with his treatment. He finds in 50% of his patients there is improvement in the myopia.

QUESTION: Don't you have to have a certain amount of Vitamin A along with your D?

DR. TAYLOR: Yes, you do. As you hear me talking today about individual vitamins which help, what I'm really assuming is that the nutritional status is such that people will have adequate amounts of all vitamins. I am up here today talking about individual vitamins helping specific conditions. But when you're talking about the eye, you're really talking about the body. The cells in the eye have their needs and the cells in the body have their needs. If you're short of something in the eye then you're going to be short of that same something in the rest of your body.

I will just say a small amount about Vitamin C. There's been enough publicity about Vitamin C so that everyone knows how important it is. Recently a physician who is in eye research at the University of Maryland seemed to feel that Vitamin C was important in helping a kind of cataract which is caused by the photochemical breakdown of oxygen in the eye to superoxide. The closest I can come to is something like ozone. Vitamin C, which is in the eye in a concentration 50-60 times greater than is found in the blood serum, is a scavenger for superoxide. You can see it is important to have plenty of ascorbic acid because, although light is extremely important to our functioning as individuals, it can present some problems, and this photochemical change in the eye is one of them. And so the Vitamin C will control that superoxide.

I don't think I really need to say much about Vitamin A. We know how Vitamin A helps in preventing night blindness. You can have a deficiency in Vitamin A in the eye even though you have adequate amounts of Vitamin A in your body. There can be plenty stored in the liver. However, if you don't have enough zinc then the protein element which carries out the distribution of Vitamin A through the body will be deficient and the Vitamin A will just sit in the liver. 50 percent of the cases of night blindness will not respond to Vitamin A until the individual gets zinc.

I've seen something in my practice related to the eye. Many patients will come to me and say their vision has been rapidly deteriorating for the past several months. They are usually wearing corrective lenses and one of the things they always ask me is: Should I go see an optometrist? I don't want to cause problems for the optometrists so I tell them not to go see their optometrist at that time because I have found that when a patient is on a good nutritional regime for a couple of months their sight begins to improve again. In the beginning I was trying to be very careful and I thought, well, if they want to see their optometrist they should go see him. And they go and they'll get some corrective lenses and then within a couple of months they are not seeing well again. Come to find out they didn't need the corrective lenses to begin with; all they had to do was to improve their nutrition.

Something else I found related to the eye is that there are some patients who do not seem able to wear contact lenses. I have one patient who has had five different contact lenses and hasn't been able to keep any of them in her eye any longer than about 15 minutes. I just want to alert you to the idea that there are some patients who are so sensitive to petrochemicals that they cannot keep lenses in their eyes, even lenses made of a gas permeable plastic. If you have a patient like that, you might suspect this kind of sensitivity. You can ask them a question which will give you a clue, and that is: Can you smell a pilot light out on a stove before anybody else in the household can? There seems to be some kind of protective mechanism with smell that if we're sensitive to something, very frequently we'll be able to smell that material more easily. If you elicit that from a patient with an affirmative answer probably 90% of the time you are dealing with a patient who has petrochemical sensitivity. A patient can also have petrochemical sensitivity and love the odor of some petrochemicals. They'll go in a gas station and they'll say, "I just love to smell that gas." One of the features of this kind of sensitivity is addiction. And so that person likes to get in that gas station and likes to smell that gasoline even though they're allergic to it. I'm going to talk a little bit more about this particular kind of allergy related to learning so you can pick up some other information that will give you a little help diagnostically.

What do you want to do for these patients? There are certain things that anybody can do to help patients when they're having vision problems. One is to just have them stop their junk foods. I have talked to a number of physicians who are in vision development and they tell me they can tell when the patients come in for their training whether they've had candy or something sweet because they don't function as well. I've also had reading specialists tell me the same thing that they know when these patients had a candy bar before coming in. Minimize alcohol ingestion because it is a carbohydrate. I'm not saying stop, I just said minimize. Stay away from hard cooking fats. Anything that's hard at room temperature really shouldn't be eaten because those little globules will get into your blood stream and they also cause clumping of cells. One of the reasons for early senility is ingestion of these hard fats causing clumping of red cells. The red cells block off the capillary; the capillaries supply 100,000 cells. So what? You've got millions of cells in your brain. If that keeps going on and on, after a period of time the cortex is going to be so riddled with scar tissue that early senility ensues, and there is no correction for something like that. The correction comes before the condition occurs.

QUESTION: Do you include butter?

Dr. TAYLOR: Yes, I include butter in that. However, butter is a little better if you'll desaturate it. There's a way of desaturating it and that's by taking one-third to one-half cup of oil–safflower oil for instance–and filling in a tablespoon full of lecithin powder. The idea of the oil in variable amounts is: How soft do you want your butter when you take it out of the icebox? The more oil you add to that butter the better off you are. But if you don't like something that drips off the knife when you try to put it on something, you may have to use a little bit less of the oil. Margarine is actually worse than butter because in order to make margarine solid, they bubble hydrogen through the oil so that about 30% of the margarine is hard fat; they're called transfats. And so margarine is not the answer, no matter what it's made from. I tell my patients to use desaturated butter if they have to have something rather than margarine.

And then you want to increase more fresh fruits, vegetables and whole grains. That is something anybody can do and most patients will accept that kind of direction from anyone. If that anyone has a degree and is in the healing area, that makes you an authority. And so if you can reach 1 out of 10 by doing that, you have accomplished a worthy goal.

This illustrates that you can't use a single vitamin to treat the eye; everything is interdependent. Look at the way all these things interrelate. Vitamin E protects Vitamin A from oxidation. When Vitamin A is depleted, Vitamin C drops. Zinc mobilizes Vitamin A via binding protein, and B5 helps promote Vitamin A production. And so you can see just giving Vitamin A is really not the ticket and there are other things that work in concert with Vitamin A. It's best the patient has all the necessary supplementation.

"You are what you eat," and that is the truth. Let me just tell you a negative aspect of things you eat. At Jefferson Medical College they found out there was a clear association between undersized anemic children and the amount of junk food fed to them at home. When they did surveys in the homes they found out that if they could find 10 junk food items or more then that child would be anemic and undersized. That an interesting correlation. In the households of the normal kids who were growing the way they were supposed to and weren't anemic, they found five or fewer junk foods in the house.

The Russians have found that nutritional supplements and amino acids, protein building blocks, are extremely important. They found out when they added supplementation and increased amino acid intake with their volunteers, that they had increased physical work capacity, better movement coordination, took less time to make decisions, and they solved arithmetical logic problems much more easily. That was a study published in 1978.

How do vitamins work? There's really not a lot of mystery about It. Vitamins are part of an enzyme system and they are coenzymes. The enzyme is a protein material and has bound to it vitamins and sometimes minerals. It's estimated there are 5,000 different enzymes in a single cell. You can see there can be quite a breakdown in the way the body functions if some of these enzymes are not put together with the proper vitamins. So if in a breakdown chain you're missing an enzyme or an enzyme which is inadequate, then you're going to have a pile up of that material, and although that material is something which may be used in the body, it can't be used, and then it becomes toxic. A lack of any of the vitamins can break an enzymatic chain so that you can have a symptom of deficiency. These deficiency signs appear slowly because the body has enzyme and vitamin reserves. Even though we don't think of water-soluble vitamins giving us reserves, they do. Take a look at these symptoms: impaired concentration, impaired attention, impaired comprehension, increased irritability. We could be talking about senility, using those symptoms, but you don't have to be senile to have these problems. You see that in people who are not nutritionally stable. You start seeing more of these symptoms in people who could be diagnosed as neurotic or even psychotic. All of those symptoms could be present before a deficiency state can be clinically diagnosed. You won't see any gross signs of vitamin or mineral deficiency, and yet have all of these symptoms. You won't find cracks at the corner of the mouth; you won't find a marble tongue, skin lesions; and yet that person walking around is vitamin and mineral deficient, and eating the standard American diet.

Back in 1947 this was proven; we've known this fact for over 30 years. And yet we still hear that you're not vitamin deficient unless you can find some kind of symptomatology in that individual. Dr. Spies did all this work in 1947. He wrote a book titled, *Rehabilitation through Better Nutrition*, and he did some very careful research. For instance, he blocked all Vitamin B1 from an individual and found all these symptoms developed and yet he could find nothing on the body to tell him that it had happened. Consider this 1968 study; eighty patients, one year duration, double blind study. Everybody likes to see a double blind study. That means if it was double blind it's a good study. 40 patients were got a placebo and 40 patients got a multi-vitamin tablet. They were photographed, checked biochemically before the study and every three months for a year. 67 of these patients showed definite signs of vitamin deficiency. Here's what happened. The patients who were on the vitamins, at 3 months 10 were improving; at 6 months 21 had improved; at 9 months 30 had improved; at 12 months 38 had improved. Of the 40 on the vitamin tablets, 38 improved. After 12 months, none of the 40 placebo patients had improved. Six were the same, 15 had worsened, 5 got much worse, and 14 had died. This shows the results of a simple multivitamin tablet. For those who had improved there was a striking difference in their general physical and mental condition. This was presented at the International Symposium on Vitamins for the Elderly in 1968, and they put this into a book called *Vitamins in the Elderly*. You can get that book and you can read it. This work was done in England. When this information was presented at that conference the American physicians said, "Things are very austere in Britain. I can imagine that happening here but not in America."

Lecture II

I'll get back to the stomach that we left before. Before you can talk too much about good nutrition, you have to make sure that the mechanisms for getting these materials into your bloodstream are working properly. If you have good teeth, able to masticate properly, and you've got saliva, that's the very first step. Next comes the stomach. Anyone over 40 should think very seriously of adding some kind of digestive to their diet. That can be done in the form of papaya. Papaya tabs can help break down the carbohydrates and start protein digestion on its way. Very possibly you might consider adding some hydrochloric acid. There are two products used: one is betaine hydrochloride which is the best. The other is glutamic acid hydrochloride. Betaine breaks down a little quicker in the stomach and doesn't carry over as much into the small intestine. You've got to be able to digest this stuff if you're going to change your diet and adding some digestives is the way to do it. The loss of digestive capability is a part of the aging process. Apparently there is a little switch in our brain that gets turned off when we're about 35-40. We're programmed apparently to live to be about 100. Anything less is related to the transgressions that we commit against ourselves.

Scientists believe that if this little switch in the brain could be found and could be influenced that the body would possibly hold up until it was 400 years old. But you're working with pretty good material if you can keep it in good shape and nutrition and vitamins and minerals are one way to keep it in good shape. But when the digestive juices start to decrease then we reduce our protein usually, and protein is the building block of the body, and so the deterioration even speeds up from that period of time.

You've got to keep a happy bowel because if you don't keep a happy bowel, then you run into the heartache of chronic constipation. Back in the 1930's intestinal poisoning was a viable kind of a theory. We believed that we absorbed toxic materials from our lower digestive tracts and then as modern medicine developed that was pooh-poohed and they said it couldn't happen. Now, believe it or not, intestinal intoxication has come full circle. It is now believed there is such a thing and I was reading recently that in the East, they have developed some testing procedures to measure the amount of end-product material that we are reabsorbing from the bowel. So you have to keep material moving through that bowel at a fairly fast clip. If you were a Bantu it would be about 14-15 hours because they get a great amount of fiber in their diet. That is something we, Americans, don't get enough of. When I'm talking about fiber I'm not talking about just any kind of fiber in foods; I'm not talking about the fiber in celery for instance. I'm talking about a very specific kind of fiber, dietary fiber. It has specific properties to it. It's thought that diverticulosis–the little pouching of the intestinal wall–is due to the fact we don't get enough fiber in our diets. If you don't have enough fiber in the diet, the bowel has to contract even harder to keep that stool moving along, and the harder it has to contract, the greater internal pressure in that bowel. With the greater pressure, the bowel starts pouching out between the muscle fibers. Once that happens then there is no changing that situation, and so it's a good idea to get a proper amount of dietary fiber before it starts happening. The most famous of dietary fiber is wheat fiber, but corn fiber and soybean husks are even better forms of fiber. Carrots are another. Dietary fiber is also a way of helping to control cholesterol. We know, of course, the effect of elevated cholesterol in the body, which is increasing the incidence of heart attacks, strokes etc.

About the American diet being adequate; more than half of the American households are deficient in one or more ways. Housewives don't have enough nutritional knowledge. It's difficult to pick proper foods in the supermarket. More and more there is not enough money for a proper diet. Since this study was done in 1965, you can see the money factor is getting worse and worse. We have problems also in the manufacturing of foods: processing is getting so complex that they're taking more and more of the good out and they leave more and more of the bad in. We're just loaded with ersatz foods. When you go out and eat in a restaurant you can almost be sure that about half of the material you get is going to be messed around with in some way.

When we talk about enrichment we're talking about adding to the beauty or quality or value or enjoyment of something. There is something we all commonly partake of which is enriched. There is a comparison of enriched white bread versus whole wheat bread. You can see the enriched bread rather than being enriched is considerably deficient in comparison with good whole wheat bread. They lost 40% of chromium in the milling, 86% of manganese, 89% of cobalt, 68% of copper, 78% of zinc, 48% of molybdenum, and this is what bread contains, the common bread that's on the market today. I used to think that bread was just made of a little salt, sugar, yeast and milk. Look at it now. The reason I'm up here making little mud balls is because this is a common loaf of white bread, enriched white bread, but can you imagine what it's like to put a lump of that in your stomach? It goes into your stomach and often does not get any further than that. Most of the bread you buy commercially, even though it says rye or wheat is primarily bleached white flour, so the nutrient value is really not good.

Here's what they do with the oil. They take that oil and run it through a filter and keep using it and using it. When you use oil for an extended period of time, especially at higher heats, it develops a toxic material called acrolein. It also gets chips of various kinds of foods in it. And so they're concerned with getting those little chips of food out and clarifying it so they can keep using it and extend its life. Some of the large places will use a filter that is similar to what you have on your filtered swimming pool with diatomaceous earth in it, and so ersatz foods are something that we're really getting loaded up with.

I'd be remiss in my duty if I didn't talk to you about sugar. Consider sugar a zero minus food. It has no food value at all. Americans are consuming about 180 pounds per capita per year and every bite of sugar that one takes costs you. That's why I say it's a zero minus food, because it takes vitamins and minerals to metabolize sugar, and so the more sugar you take; the shorter you get on vitamins. Sugar has all kinds of deleterious biochemical effects also. It interferes with calcium/phosphorous ratio. Within 10 minutes after eating sugar the calcium and phosphorous ratio begins to reverse itself in the body. This is not as much a problem with adults as it is with children. Increasing phosphorous tends to make children more hyper because phosphorous is a mineral which increases activity. Not only is that occurring but you're interfering with that child's growth. It also interferes with phagocytic index. It diminishes the ability of the phagocytes in the blood stream to fight infection.

We do have malnutrition in this country. The state of nutrition is such that it's estimated in a recent study that 2 million children per year are being born with learning difficulties because the mothers were undernourished during pregnancy. Early under-nutrition equals a small head and a small head equals a small brain. These are mothers who get approximately 70% of the full requirement of carbohydrate and about 40% of the full requirement for protein. One of the few things that the *Journal of the American Medical Association* has published is in relation to this malnutrition in general medical patients.

Here there were three single nutritional surveys at weekly intervals with 251 patients. They checked height, weight, triceps, skin fold, arm circumferences, serum albumin, the percentage of red cells to plasma, lymphocytes, and they computed the nutrient intake on a weekly basis. 44% were considered to have protein calorie deficiency. These people had low albumins. Here is the same thing at the University of Alabama Medical School. One hundred medical-surgical patients hospitalized two weeks or more; two-thirds lost weight in the hospital, and this wasn't because of their condition.

One-half had low serum albumin levels, but only two-thirds of them had a correction made. One-fifth became anemic in the hospital and one-fourth had evidence of vitamin depletion but no vitamins prescribed. Hospitals are not the safest place a person can go for good nutrition.

If you just go out and take a generalized survey of people for vitamin deficiencies, you'll find that anyone who isn't paying attention to good nutrition or taking some kind of vitamin therapy is going to have some kind of vitamin deficiency. Dr. Babcock several years ago went to Pittsburgh and surveyed so-called healthy iron workers who have a good income; they can afford good food, and about 20% of them had a Vitamin C deficiency and 25% of them were low in B1. These were just random samplings. And so I don't think you can say the American diet is an adequate diet.

Talking a little bit about learning disability, here's a brain, composed of billions of cells, it weighs approximately 3 pounds and yet requires 25% of all available nutrition to the body. If we just had some inkling of what really goes on in the brain we'd go a long way to correcting a lot of the problems that we see more and more. Learning disabilities are on the upswing. In talking to 1st, 2nd, and 3rd grade teachers, they tell me that their referrals to the school psychologist increase every single year. I think you could say without fear of contradiction that a lot of that has to do with nutrition. These kids don't come to school with breakfast many times, or if they do they have eaten some sugar-coated kind of cereal, and they don't have anything to work with and sugar creates all kinds of problems, for instance, changing the calcium-phosphorous ratio in the brain. It also plays a great part in central nervous system allergy which I'll mention.

It looks like they're getting a little closer to finding out something about hyperactivity. Here's something very recent, talking about neural transmitters in the brain which are protein and vitamin dependent and an attempt to classify hyperactivity according to neural transmitter imbalances. Serotonin is a calming transmitter. Catecholamines are excitatory transmitters. This results in the following four classifications: a normal serotonin with excessive catecholamine, low serotonin and excessive catecholamines, low serotonin and normal catecholamines and then excessive amounts of both. Serotonin at certain levels is a calmer, but when it gets too high then serotonin becomes an excitatory transmitter. When the person took the glass of milk just before going to bed to help them sleep–and it did help some people sleep–it was because of the essential amino acid in milk, tryptophan. Tryptophan can raise serotonin. But if you want to be sure you don't cause troubles, you also have to make sure that Vitamin B6 and niacinamide are there also, because if serotonin is not broken down further, then you can develop a problem with excessive amounts of serotonin and get a hyper individual. B6 and niacinamide are essential when tryptophan is given. Ascorbic acid also helps to raise serotonin. Ascorbic acid is a mono amine oxidase inhibitor and mono amine oxidase destroys serotonin in the brain. Even foods can affect serotonin. If you have a carbohydrate meal serotonin is increased so that you have an increased sensitivity to pain, you're sleepier and you can have a reduced appetite. This was one of the ideas of eating a little candy before a meal. It can raise serotonin. Feeling sleepy 15-20 minutes after having a meal can also be related to having your serotonin increased. If the protein is increased that will drive the serotonin down: insomnia, exaggerated sexual activity, and so you can take your choice between manipulating carbohydrate and protein.

At the University of Winnipeg, Department of Psychology, they had a group of children who had learning disabilities with soft neurological signs, balance difficulties, poor visual or auditory discrimination. They had problems; they confused right and left. These kids were given niacinamide, B6, and ascorbic acid for a period of time and after that administration of these materials their learning difficulties began to decrease. One thing I want to point out about working with learning disabilities, nutrition, vitamins and minerals is that good nutrition, vitamins and minerals will help the individual learn, but you still have to train the individual. Two things must go hand in hand: You have to train as well as improve the biochemical substrate. One or the other won't get the job done. That old mythology about fish being brain food is not mythology any longer. Fish has a lot of choline in it. The choline is converted into another neurotransmitter in the brain called acetyloholine and at MIT about a year ago it was discovered that choline is the most important vitamin related to memory. There's been a product on the market since the late 1950's called Deaner. It is just choline that's been modified so it will pass the blood brain barrier. Sometimes choline in smaller amounts will help memory but if you take it in larger amounts then you get tremendous odor and no one wants to be around you. Lecithin, for instance, contains a moderate amount of choline.

Zinc is the smart mineral, because its part of the enzyme system in the brain and it enhances learning. As I mentioned before, zinc is probably the most common mineral deficiency today, because we just don't get it in our foods any longer, but zinc is just tremendously important because it has anti-allergy effects. It is part of the immunological system helping us resist infections; helps hair grow; helps to control acne in teenagers. It's part of the anti-stress system. Within 15 minutes after some severe stress the zinc will begin showing up in the urine, indicating that it's used apparently to detoxify some of the materials developed during a stressful situation. It's especially important to the male because if you have inadequate zinc your testosterone level is going to decrease. Testosterone is the hormone that gives us our zip and our push and our drive, but it' is also important in protein metabolism and controls protein metabolism. Many cases of infertility on the part of the male are related to having low zinc.

It would be interesting to see how many in this audience can detect a possible zinc deficiency in themselves. This is one thing you may be able to detect before it becomes too severe. Everyone should take a look at their nails right now and see if there are any white spots or streaks on their nails. If you don't mind, I'd like to see how many of you can find some white spots on their nails. A white spot on the nail is not due to a trauma; it's a zinc deficiency. About a fifth of you raised your hands, and if you're males, you're in trouble especially because another important factor relating to zinc is that the prostate requires zinc in order to operate properly. If it doesn't have the zinc it will begin to swell, hypertrophy. At the University of Illinois Medical School about a year ago–this was up in Chicago–they had approximately 400 male patients who were to have prostate surgery. They gave those 400 patients zinc for two months. That was the only thing they gave them as an added supplementation. At the end of two months 300 of those 400 patients did not have to have surgery. That's a simple way to avoid having a surgical procedure on your prostate. They used zinc sulphate and I'm not enthusiastic about zinc sulphate. I like other types of zinc; I like zinc gluconate better. The minimum daily requirement for a male or any human being is 15 mg. per day. I'd advise a minimum of twice that per day, and that should be a ritual for the rest of your life because you're not going to get it in the food; you're not going to get it in the grain or the meat or the vegetables! It's a very simple way to avoid the statistic that one out of every four American males has his prostate taken out. It seems to be related to zinc intake doesn't it?

Dr. Cott, a psychiatrist in New York, published some results of treating 500 learning disabled children, using vitamins and mineral supplementation with very good general improvement in almost all of these kids. Lead is bad stuff. I don't know if you have problems with lead up here, but in Los Angeles just the smog is enough to increase lead content in children. One of the things that help to control lead is zinc. Here are these kids not getting enough zinc and they have all this lead floating around in the smog the air. Smog has been falling for so long that in many areas of Los Angeles the ground is literally coated with lead dust, and the smaller the child, the more lead exposure they get because they're running around kicking up that dust and they're low enough to the ground to breathe that lead dust in. I found with hair analyses I really don't have to know where the child is from. If the child comes from my county, which is Ventura County where there is a minimum amount of smog, they generally do not have very high lead levels, but if they come from Los Angeles they almost universally have elevated lead. Lead tends to reduce the intelligence quotients of kids–knocks off about 10 points from an IQ Test score–and you have these soft neurological signs, and I find that a very high percentage of the hyperactive children I see have high lead levels, therefore it probably contributes to hyperactivity also.

As a little sidelight, obsessive-compulsive seems to respond to tryptophan. Apparently low tryptophan levels can cause obsessive-compulsive behavior. In a report that was published this year by the Nassau Mental Health Clinic's Yayura Tobias, they got improvement in 90% of obsessive-compulsives by using tryptophan, B6 and niacinamide, the formula I outlined before. Treating an obsessive-compulsive patient with psychotherapy is virtually impossible. Whenever they get an improvement in obsessive-compulsive behavior with psycho therapy they write it up in a journal because it's so unusual. Here it looks as if obsessive compulsive behavior is linked, to a certain degree, to something going on biochemically in the individual.

B15 is another interesting vitamin or non-vitamin depending on who you listen to. B15 is an oxygenator. It was first used by the Russians in treating non-verbal children, children who are late talkers. B15 seemed to be excellent in treating non-verbal children. Also it seemed to be very helpful in treating children who verbalize to a minimum degree. Give them B15 and the verbalization is noticeably increased in these kids. Also, because it's an oxygenator, I give it to all the athletes I treat and they report improved performances after they've been taking it for a short while, especially the runners. Pangamic acid is another name for B15.

This is Anna Thompson. She has central nervous system allergy. Anna Thompson was being tested using a technique of putting drops of food extract under her tongue and then observing what went on. You can see that she started out pretty well. Right where the arrow is we gave her sugar under the tongue, and you can see what happened. She just went bananas. We've been able to demonstrate reversals with this technique. The kid will be riding along just beautifully and will be given an allergen under the tongue and they'll start doing reversals. You give them a neutralizing dose and the reversals stop. This kind of allergy has a very powerful effect on the central nervous system. Some people call it getting brain hives, but the brain apparently does swell when you ingest something you're allergic to. Probably 60% of the population in this room have central nervous system allergy. The primary site of action is the brain and then it causes other systemic problems. Some researchers believe, for instance, that diabetes is actually an allergic problem and they have demonstrated, as have I, that when you give a full blown diabetic a carbohydrate that they are not allergic to, their blood sugar will only go up slightly, but you give them a food they are allergic to, a carbohydrate for instance, and their blood sugar will just shoot out of sight. They'll be running along at maybe a 200; you give them wheat, and if they're allergic to it, their blood sugar can pop up to 380-400. You give them corn; and they're not allergic to it, their blood sugar will not change in sublingual testing. The same can be demonstrated by having them ingest food.

This kind of allergy is hidden or masked because the symptoms of the allergy are not what you expect. It's not the itchy eye, runny nose, wheezy, kind of an allergy, although it can cause those symptoms. Once you eat a food you're allergic to, the allergy symptoms can last for 3-5 days. These kinds of allergies are related primarily to the foods we commonly have in our diet. If you're allergic to wheat, for instance, and you have wheat every day of the week, it's almost impossible to avoid it. You're never free of this kind of allergy. I can say that I've never examined a hyperactive child who does not have central nervous system allergy. How great of a component the central nervous system allergy is to the hyperactivity, I don't know, but it's always there in these children.

QUESTION: Will taking B6 with the wheat help?

DR. TAYLOR: If you take Vitamin B6 orally, and take some wheat, it probably will not help. If you give Vitamin B6 intravenously after somebody has ingested an allergen, then it's quite possible you can knock out the allergic reaction. The other thing that causes tremendous problems in these central nervous system allergy people are petroleum petrochemicals. Food dyes are petrochemicals, and so this is probably the basis for a lot of children having hyperactivity related to food dyes. But you can't demonstrate this in all children and the sublingual testing helps to differentiate these food dye reactors from non-food dye reactors, and of course learning difficulties are greatly enhanced by this kind of allergy.

There are some ways you can recognize these people when they come into the office. One of the ways is by looking at their 5th finger, and if you find that the finger curves in, toward the midline, to any great extent, you are beginning to establish the fact that they are probably allergic kids with this kind of allergy. Another thing that you notice is an incomplete Palmer Line. This line is called the Heart Line by Palmer. It generally should go up without breaking up close between these two fingers. If it's foreshortened and you have an incurved little finger, you can almost stop right there. You've got a kid with central nervous system allergy or an adult with the same. Also, the eyes are a giveaway because the eyes are usually dark underneath and a little bit puffy, and the inner corners are opened up. The upper and lower lids don't kiss in the midline. When you see that you are dealing with someone who has central nervous system allergy, a lot of their behaviors and their difficulties become related. In sublingual testing we can turn visual problems on and off, visual acuity on and off, by giving them something they're allergic to and then giving them a neutralizing dose. Visual acuity can decrease for several hours after having a food to which the person is allergic. In the history you'll almost always find out that this child or this adult had some feeding problems: vomiting, formula changing. Milk allergy in the child almost always causes ear problems. If you get a history of a child who had a number of earaches, or an adult who can remember having earaches, it's probably–in my practice anyway–95% sure that they have a milk allergy. One of the mythologies about this kind of allergy is that you grow out of it. You don't grow out of it. You stop having rashes; you stop vomiting; you stop having earaches; it just takes another form. It goes underground so that you will have difficulty in learning to read or behavioral problems.

Just recognizing the possibility of a milk allergy can create some miraculous cures. Kids walking around with the ear tubes because they had frequent earaches, when you get them off of milk and milk products for two weeks, you'd be amazed. This is something that anybody can do. The central nervous system allergy plays a big part in learning disabilities in general physical problems of both children and adults.

QUESTION: Can you tell us more about the diagnosis of central nervous system allergy related to the eyelids?

DR. TAYLOR: Usually the eyelid in the midline of both lids will meet or kiss, but in the person with central nervous system allergy the inner angle is widened and probably because there is some pressure on both upper and lower lid, forcing them outward so that they roll up and down. When you see that, then you've got a pretty good idea if it matches up with some of these other things.

I'm just going to mention some B12, and as I'm mentioning B12 I'm going to start putting a bibliography up here. These are things I'd recommend that you obtain. The *Nutrition Almanac* is a good little book to have. A psychiatrist in New York City, H. L. Newbold, has found that 33% of the patients he sees have B12 deficiencies or very low B12. He wrote *Meganutrients for Your Nerves*, a very good book to get for your reference material. A couple of years ago we had a big scare because a Dr. Herbert said that ascorbic acid interfered with the ability of B12 to work in the body. That is still being taught now. A PhD in nutrition at UCLA, her name is Alfyn Slater, is still telling all her students that ascorbic acid destroys Vitamin B12 in the body. It's starting to appear in textbooks now. This whole thing has been debunked. That result came because of a faulty lab technique, and it didn't help any because Dr. Herbert happens to be one of the physicians who believes it's not necessary to take vitamins, and so it carried more weight and it was picked up by the news services, medical science writers on newspapers because this is the kind of information they get The FDA is interested in controlling all vitamins. They want to make vitamins by prescription only, and so every time they come up with a study indicating that vitamins are detrimental it goes to all of the medical news writers and science editors of all the major newspapers in the US. But major newspapers are reluctant to cover meetings which deal with nutrition if it is sponsored by an organization like International College of Applied Nutrition because it's not party line. The FDA failed once in trying to get vitamins on prescription and they're building up to this again. And so if one person in 180 million people would have a Vitamin A poisoning, you'd be sure to hear about it.

If you have a person who is a Vitamin B12 deficient, of course, it interferes with energy production in the body. The B12 has to be given in very large amounts because there are certain people who are B12 dependent individuals, meaning they have to have larger amounts of B12 than the normal individual, and you can give them a normal amount of B12 and nothing happens. When their tissues finally get saturated with B12, it's like someone has turned the key on; all of a sudden they just pick up. I see this demonstrated time and time again in my office because in my office I load them up by giving it to them by injection and within two weeks there is a vast, vast difference in these people.

Mental and Elemental Nutrients is a tremendous book by Carl Pfeiffer PhD MD. *Vitamins and Hormones* is a very handy little reference to have around. Ross Flume Hall, *Food for Naught* is a nutritional researcher and his particular thing is the way foods have lost their quality of nutrition by processing. It's a very excellent book to read. I want to recommend one more book to you before I close because it shows the continued recognition of the part that diet plays in behavior. This is a fairly new book out. It's called *How to Improve your Child's Behavior through Diet* by Laura J. Stevens, Rosemary B. Stoner and it's a Doubleday. It talks a great deal about the relationship of allergy to behavior and has lots of recipes in it. It's worth getting as a reference because you can tell a mother how to make little goodies for their children that don't have sugar in them.

QUESTION: What are good sources of zinc?

DR. TAYLOR: A zinc tablet. Zinc sulphate is not good. Zinc gluconate is the best.

QUESTION: What foods contain zinc?

DR. TAYLOR: Beef contains zinc; grains contain zinc; and some green leafies contain zinc. If you can get the foods grown in ground that has zinc in it, and also if you can get food which has not had artificial fertilizer used on it, then you are likely to get an adequate zinc intake.

QUESTION: How do you find a referral source?

DR. TAYLOR: I don't know. It depends on where you're from. I know that in Seattle there are a couple of people who do work in this area. I can't tell you their names. I don't know about Portland and I don't know about other areas in the Pacific Northwest.

I hope that today maybe I've been able to scare you just a little bit and to get you out of your complacency and believing that what you are eating is adequate, because it definitely is not. The information available confirms that it is not and the information is now starting to come from medical school research, so you can feel safe in believing it. Thank you.

Dr. Irving Borish
Vectographic Techniques for Binocular Refraction
1982

During the course of working with these clinical methods of various types, some years back I came to realize that when we talk about modern refractive techniques in modern optometry that in a sense we were flattering our egos, not always legitimately because most of the things we do in optometry are quite old from the standpoint of scientific advancement. In fact, we are only introducing in some ways some techniques that actually are very, very old and just haven't been used. For example, we like to think that if we have a modern unit with a refractor, keratometer and even a slit lamp and a good retinoscope and ophthalmoscope that we're pretty well equipped and we're doing a pretty competent job. Some of you have heard me read these figures off but I'll do them again

The ophthalmoscope, 1851. Ophthalmometer, the first 1854. Later than that, Javal-Schiotz's, 1884. Perimeter, 1801. The arc perimeter, 1869. Let's take the photo keratoscope, 1896. The slit lamp, the illumination system was developed in 1911. The microscope in 1897. The combined slit lamp in 1916. Retinoscope, 1861. Snellen test chart, 1362. Green clock dial, 1867. Jackson Cross Cylinder, 1887 to 1893; Jackson described the technique in great detail in 1901, but Donders described it in 1850 under a different name.

The real new inventions are automatic refraction. That is a real radical change in technique. We haven't learned how to handle that yet. But there are techniques in between that exist that many of us haven't even attempted; some of us have. We're finding now that what we're putting into our clinics are things like photo-slit lamps. There are two unique techniques in the literature and we're just now learning how to use one of them, and one has been out a little while but we haven't used it widely. One is binocular refraction. The other technique is fixation disparity as a diagnostic method. We're just as traditionally locked in to the old phorias and ductions and blur points that Sheard first described as a routine in 1921 in the American Journal of Physiology Optics. We're still locked into that after 60 years. We find ourselves very slow in accepting changes in our methodologies, concepts and our thinking, in our instrumentation and in our procedures.

I'm going to talk to you now about binocular refraction. What do we mean by binocular refraction? We mean the difference between occluding one eye in its entire perceptual field while I examine the other eye and having that eye open; exposed and seeing while I examine the other eye. To do that, obviously something in my target must make it so that I can identify that it is this eye that is responding. Why do binocular refraction? One of the things I've tried to bring to you is that if we're going to make some propositions we're going to show you some figures. We have taken patients and done the routine with monocular refraction and done the routine with binocular refraction, and seeing whether there is any difference and if it's statistically significant. One of the things we find in binocular refraction of value is that there is a difference in endpoint. What do I mean by endpoint? I mean the place where you decide to stop the subjective. With one qualification – the place where you decide to stop the subjective is the interpretation that this is the best acuity, the best focus you can get. You may decide to stop the subjective in some other place for some other reason, but that is a discretionary choice. This is the place for the best lens for the best acuity. There is a difference of whether you cover this eye or whether you expose both eyes. That difference shows to various extents. 20-35% of the subjects tested will show a difference of +/- 0.25D. However, 2-12% will show as much of a difference of as much as +/- 0.50 and others show some differences as high as +/- 2.50D. And so you do find a difference even in the endpoint when you do binocular refraction. If we take the Turville Method and if we do it with a Haploscope which is the best method we have of determining when the image is actually focused exactly on the retina, we find it agrees within +/- 0.25D in the main with binocular refraction, then we get better equalization

Let me explain something about equalization. Too many people get the impression that when we talk of equalization what we're talking about is equalization of vision and what we actually mean is not equalization of vision at all. We use vision for the purpose of equalizing but what we're equalizing has nothing to do with vision. What then do I mean by equalization? What I mean is equalization of accommodative effort. I want the two eyes to accommodate together. You can't accommodate one eye without the other. Consequently, if he is to adopt a hyperopic posture here and zero there, and he looks at that chart, if he has this eye in focus he is going to have to be a diopter out of focus here. There is no way he can be using both eyes together, and that is even more so when he looks at near. And so if I don't equalize him correctly at far, I'm going to wind up with a pair of eyes that are not really getting the same clarity of images on both retinas and I have a problem in fusion.

Now what we do want to do is to equalize as exactly as we can. What do we find? We find that if we equalize under binocular perceptual systems as compared to monocular ones, 25% of our patients will show a difference in equalization of +/- 0.25D over what they showed before whereas over 6% will show as much as +/- 0.50D difference. That is an important aspect in the average accommodative equalization,

Let me point out something to you. Here is the vertical meridian of my right eye. Here is the vertical meridian of my left eye. If I want to fuse they must be parallel. What do you do? Let's assume for the sake of argument I have a slight cyclophoria of my right eye of 10°. Now you sit me in your refracting chair and you say, "We will test your right eye," and we close this eye. What did you suppose happens to this eye? It goes into the cyclophoric position automatically. It goes into the cyclophoric position. Now you do a very careful refraction and you come up with +3.00 -1.50 x 105, and now you open the other eye And so you give me the glasses and I go out and I come back a week later and I say, "I can't tell you what's the matter but there's something about these glasses that bothers me." How much do you find in cyclophoria? We find an average of 8.0° of change and a change of 10° in at least 2% of the cases. The cylinder axis will change by that much when you do binocular refraction as compared to monocular refraction. What happens if you don't put a prism in and I come down and try to fuse? It's going to change axis, right? What happens if you do put a prism in? You are going to let me take the cyclophoric position and it makes a difference in what you're going to do with your cylinder as to whether you put a prism in or not.

Now let me tell you about eccentric fixation. Many years ago I came here to Pacific to lecture to the students and they heard I could do a routine very quickly. They said, "If we set a chair up will you do it in front of our class?" And so they dragged a chair out and they pulled a student into the chair. Of course, I had been with students many years and so I knew that probably I was looking at a +4.00 - 5.00 x 130, but I refracted the patient and went through the routine for them

Now this is one of the first things that Turville discovered. Here is a patient looking at a binocular refraction chart. He sees the frame of the chart; he sees the septum with both eyes; he sees the 1 with his one eye and lo and behold he is fusing the frame; he is fusing the septum and the 2 letters are out of line vertically. Turville called this a vertical phoria because he didn't know anything about vertical disparity. We know today that this is really a measure of vertical disparity. What we discovered was the prism which corrected that was wearable by the patient. Of all the vertical methods of trying to prescribe the right vertical prism, the best one turned out to be the Turville Test or binocular test. We can also do this laterally. Unfortunately, the prism prescribed from this is not always wearable, but it does give us some indication that something is haywire. It permits measuring aniseikonia and stereo acuity. All these things can be done by binocular refractive methods.

How do we get binocular refraction? The simplest method is the physical septum like the Turville one, or Morgan's on a projector, or Louis Jaques did it at the near-point many years ago with a septum along the reading rod. Here is the Turville Method. There is the chart behind the patient's eyes; there is the mirror in front with the septum. The left eye will see the "L"; the right eye will see the "F" in the mirror, but if you trace the "L" you'll notice it hits the septum and so it never gets into the right eye. And so both eyes see the frame of the mirror; both see the septum but only one sees the "L" and one sees the "F", and so I can test either eye separately while both eyes are fusing together. Morgan developed this into a projection system. Why didn't it become popular in the US? Because we like to use projectors and we didn't like mirrors and charts. Morgan developed a slide which had 2 charts at such a separation that if you placed the septum halfway between the patient and the chart, you could produce the same effect. The problem with Morgan's Method was the patient always walked into the septum and you had to remeasure and reset it and it was a nuisance. If I was doing it again today I would have one of these wall tracks such as they put studio lights in, and move my septum along that track. It is an adaptation of Turville. Where Turville had the mirror at the septum point and the chart back here, here you have the chart down there. Other types of septums are psychological ones. In other words, you can blur the untested eye. Unfortunately, that doesn't tell you everything the septum system does.

The methods we use today are polarization and let me explain those to you. Polaroid is a system whereby we confine the vibrations of light to a given plane and if we had two Polaroid's in synchrony the light will get through, and if we them at right angles to each other the light will not get through. We have three ways of polarizing. One is to overlay the entire field, the other is to polarize the letters only, and the third is to use a Vectograph. Originally we overlaid the entire field. Titmus even made a test procedure like that which was not successful. Polaroid charts were first designed by Dartmouth people when they worked with aniseikonia. Then there was Norman with overlay, Frantz with a colored background, Grolman with a Vectograph, and Eskridge with a Vectograph and a background. Now you can see there is an "F" and an "L" up there you're supposed to be looking at and this is the retina. What you get is this: the "F" is put on as a black letter on a polarized field in one direction, the "L" is on a as a black letter on a whole polarized field in the other direction. You put a piece of Polaroid that matches the polarization directions in front of each eye so the light from the background on the "F" side comes through on the right eye but it won't come through on the left eye so the left eye will see a black field. The "L", the Polaroid runs this way and the filter runs this way so the length from the background will get through on the left side but the right side coming through will form a black field. So the right side sees a black "F" on a white field with the other letter is blacked out, the left side sees a black letter "L" on a white field while the other side is blacked out. If you do this in a lighted room the two black fields can be

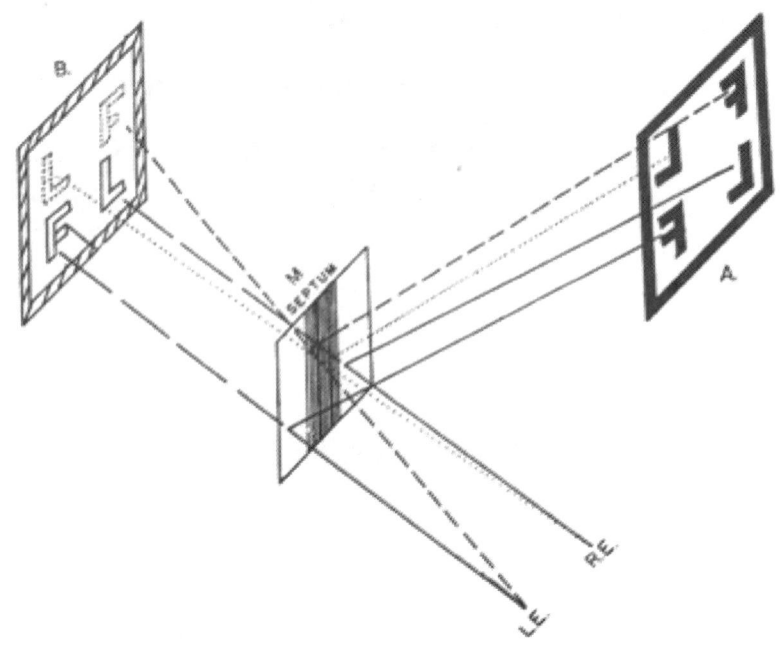

Figure 1: This figure is from Borish, Clinical Refraction, and page 758 of the third edition (1975). "A" is the actual test chart on the wall above and behind where the patient is seated. The markings "L.E." and "R.E." refer to the patients left and right eyes correspondingly. "M" is the object that appears before the patient with a septum in the middle and mirrors on either side through which the patients sees the target "A". What the patient sees is the projected image "B".

fused, but if you do it in a dark room the two black fields blend in the background and you have two independent fields, which are not really fused.

We have a problem here. The letters are polarized, but the background is not. You and I are talking about projecting these letters on a screen We have been unable to find enough artists who can engrave the Lord's Prayer on the head of a pin to attach the Polaroid to the 20/15, 20/20, and 20/30 letters on a slide. You realize what a mechanical problem that would be. It is too expensive to make and so that has held us up There we were, we knew if we could get this Polaroid we could get this thing really working and yet we couldn't do it until the vectographic slide was developed. Now how does the vectograph work? Dichroic crystals are a special kind of crystal which on a stretched polyvinyl alcohol film will transmit light only along one axis and will absorb it in the other axis. In other words, if

204

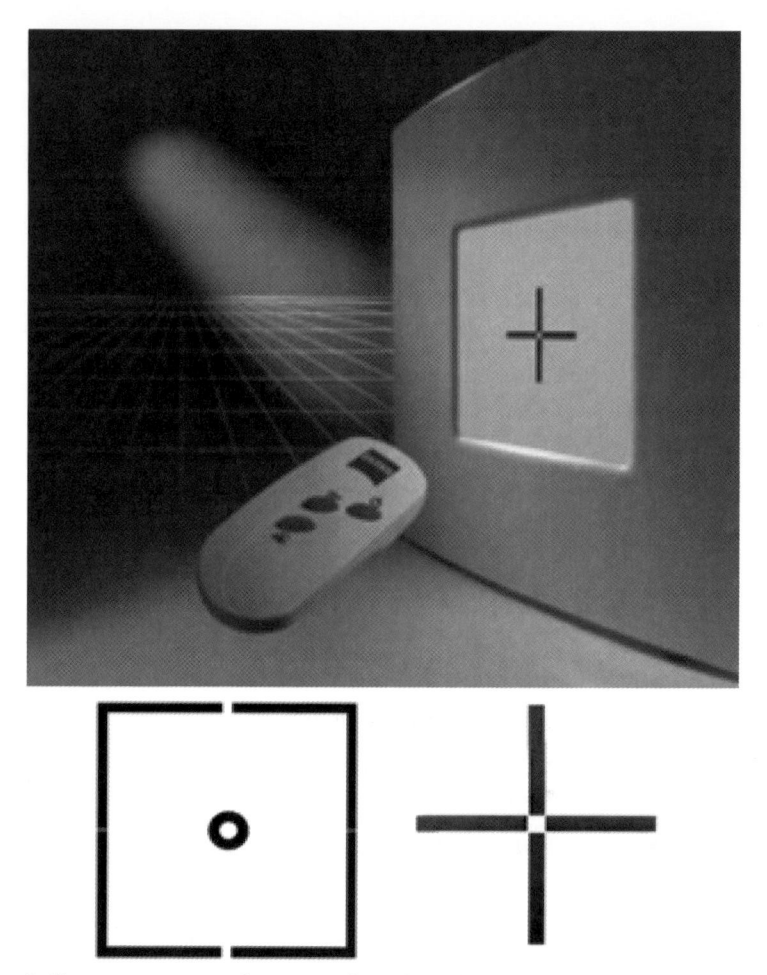

Figure 2: Here are some sample pictures from the Pola test that is made by Zeiss. It is a distance projected Polaroid set of several targets, only two of which are shown here, that can be used as described in the text. In the figure on the left the circle is seen by both eyes but each of the bracket figures are seen by only one eye. In the figure on the right, one vertical bar and one horizontal bar are seen by each eye with only the screen and wall being seen with both eyes.

you get a bunch of crystals on a film and you stretch the film, all the crystals will line up the same way, and it's the same as if you got a piece of Polaroid. They actually absorb and then readmit the light. Those crystals can be made into an ink, and so if we print the symbol on dichroic crystal dye it will transmit light just like the background, and, in other words, I can make an ink with which I can print, and if I can print I can print small letters. So that's how the vectograph was developed into the final chart.

How does it work? In this case I drew the line in both directions to indicate the light is coming in both directions. We put the analyzers opposite to the screen and, lo and behold, the F goes through the screen—doesn't go through and it looks black; the background, ½ of it goes through the screen and it looks white so you have a black letter on a white background. The other side, ½ the background goes through the screen but so does the L and so the other side just looks blank white Now don't take the entrance vision without Polaroid. You are having your patient look at grey letters. Put the Polaroid in front of their old Rx because you must make the letter black and the only way you can do it is with the filter with the analyzer. Whether or not he sees as well as he would have seen on your other chart isn't important because that's another one of these fallacies. It doesn't matter. Suppose they do see better on one chart than the other. That's not the point. The point is what's the best they see on the chart I'm using when they come in, what's the best they see when I send them out? Those are the two things I have to compare. But if you want black letters you have to use the Polaroid

The next test Grofman thought of as a phoria test, but now he does not know what it is and none of the rest of us knows either. [1] Theoretically, it is supposed to be a phoria test but you can't take a phoria when you fuse peripherally. The next chart with the little circle and dot is a disparity test and it also includes a form of a stereo acuity test. But there is one thing we all forget and I think we all forget our elementary optics. The first law we all learned in optics was the law which said the angle of incidence equals the angle of reflection. I have had innumerable men over the country say to me, "Yes, I tried using the vectograph but it's so dim." I said, "Draw me your room," and they would draw it for me. Most rooms are something like this. The projector is over on one side, or it's on the unit, or it's up above the chair if they're using these remote control projectors. If you follow this one, we went in and we took a mirror from a lady's purse and we cemented it and stuck it on the chart, and we turned the room perfectly dark, and we lit the projector and we looked for where the reflection was, and we discovered that if our patient would be sitting near the ceiling in the next room that we would have a bright image. In other words, when you put in the Polaroid, the Polaroid cuts 50%

---

1. *Editors Note: This type of testing emerged in two forms to be called either "fixation disparity" testing or tests of "associated phorias".*

to begin with and you've lowered the illumination intensity so much that that chart looks dim. You want a bright chart with a vectograph. Put it on a universal joint or put it on a hinge, tilt it a little and you can have the brightest chart you want, and don't excuse yourself if you have a remote control chart above the patient's head because the patient's eyes are not in their feet because you are going to bounce the other way just the same. You have to balance it both ways. The universal joint is the best way. If you do that you'll get a very bright vectographic target back at the refractor. You won't find this a bad decision to modify your projection setup this way.

Do you know why I use this chart? I don't know of any other to use. I have gone to every manufacturer and asked, "Why don't you make binocular instrumentation?" I was at Bausch & Lomb a whole day a couple of years ago talking about instrument improvement. They called me recently when they came out with their new refractor and I said, "Does it have Polaroid in it?" "No." "Do you have any kind of vectographic binocular slide?" "No." They just don't do it. What can you do? You can adapt the slide. You can get that glass part out of the slide and adapt it to whatever slide will fit in your projector. But I think if we all put enough pressure on the different manufacturers they will suddenly wake up to the date.

We can also introduce a better near-point analysis and I want to show you some factors of the near-point analysis that you might add to the elements you are already dealing with. Most of us test our near-point on the primary plane of sight, the reading route. I do the same as you do but I want to bring home to you the factor that this set of tests is not as critical as you and I would like it to be. The average individual, if he looks through the optical centers of his lenses, even if he converges a little to the side, is no longer looking through the optical power of those lenses as they are truly expressed because the true power is a function of where they are looking relative to the optical center. One of the things we do is we test the distance vision on a primary plane and I test phorias etc. in the same position. I want to point out the classical von Graefe phoria test which we all use and which is probably the most popular phoria test made is the test in which I place a vertical prism in front of one eye and drop a chart in space, and a base in prism in front of the other eye, and move it over to one side. Now I have two charts like that with prism in front of my eye and I ask the patient to tell me either when those charts become level or aligned one above the other one. One of the things that the phoria discloses to us physiologically is the amount of fusional convergence being used to see singly That is, that fusional convergence in use that is independent of accommodation; consequently, to measure it, accommodation must be locked. That means we must be sure the accommodation stays constant while we perform the test. Why? Because if we allow the accommodation to increase, if we allow it to decrease, we will be introducing or changing the amount of accommodative convergence involved, and then our test will vary and it won't be telling us that convergence that is free of accommodation, which is what the test should tell us.

Here's another problem. Here is a chart down here and out here. I want to ask you, what is the action of the medial rectus of the eye and the lateral rectus when the eyes are in the primary position? We all know that. The medial rectus turns the eye in and the lateral rectus turns the eye out. What is the action of the medial or lateral rectus muscles when I am declining 40°? They no longer just turn the eye either in and out; they have other actions as well. They do vertical and torsional things to it when I'm looking 40° down. What is the action of the superior rectus when the eye is looking straight ahead? It turns the eye up and pulls it in. What is the action of the superior rectus when the eye turns to the right a given number of degrees? It then purely elevates. What about the oblique with the eye straight ahead, or down, or out, etc.? And so, I change the whole muscle action with the two charts. Which one shall I have them look at? If he looks at the lower one I change it in one direction and if he looks at the right one I change it in the other direction. I may be measuring something but I'm not measuring the position of the balance of the eyes in the primary position. This is not a good test. We don't know what it tells us but it's simple and easy to take. Who wants to bother with a Maddox Rod anyway? And so we continue with it.

Let's check these things. Accommodation varies with the error. Let me take you through an elemental exercise in optics. I used a very strong lens here. Plano light strikes a -10.00D lens and leaves the back surface of the lens at a -10.00D wave and it moves through a vertex distance of 15mm and it becomes -8.69D and focuses on that retina. The wave comes up now, it's already a -2.50D when it hits the front of the lens and so it goes through the lens and so it now is at -12.50D. Now as it moves down to the cornea it's a -10.53D, but only -8.69D is going to focus on his retina and so he has to accommodate +1.84D. A -10.00D myope looking at near only accommodates +1.84D to see clearly.

Let's take a +10.00D hyperope. It takes a +10.00D lens on the front, goes out on a back at a +10.00D wave, and by the time it hits the eye it's a +11.75D and that's what focuses on the retina. Let's have him look at 40 centimeters. It comes up as a -2.50D, leaves as a +7.50D, and by the time it hits the eye it's +8.43D, and it's +3.33D to divergence and he has to accommodate, and so the myope of 10D accommodates 1.83D and the hyperope of 10D accommodates 3.33D! You and I like to think that whatever the refractive error is, we put spectacles on him out here at 14-15mm from his eye and from now on when he looks at 40 centimeters he's going to accommodate 2.50D. It just isn't so. Consequently in anisometropia of any extent, I have two entirely different accommodative demands than I thought I had even though I think I've equalized the vision at far.

Can we work this out without having to go through these drawings? Yes, you can use Joseph Pascal's old accommodative unit.[2] You young fellows don't know Joseph Pascal. Go to your library and you'll see a book by Pascal. If you want to read more on this subject, take that book home and read it. It consists of the lectures he used to give when he was teaching ophthalmology and optometry at Columbia University. He developed what he called the accommodative unit. What is it? It's the accommodation for the error that can be determined by the accommodative unit for any given error. How do you determine it? It is 1-0.03(D)=AUM The D stands for the amount of myopia For my 10D myope it would be 1-0.03*(10). That equals 1-0.3=0.7. That is how much the accommodative unit is for the 10D myope. What is his working distance? 40 cms = 2.50D x 0.7=1.75D. It is this lens effectivity difference that explains why corrective hyperopes frequently run into presbyopia earlier than corrected myopes.

---

2. Pascal JI. *(Department of Ophthalmology, N. Y. Polyclinic Medical School and Hospital)* Basis and Applications of the Accommodative Unit, Ophthalmologica 1950;120:428-434

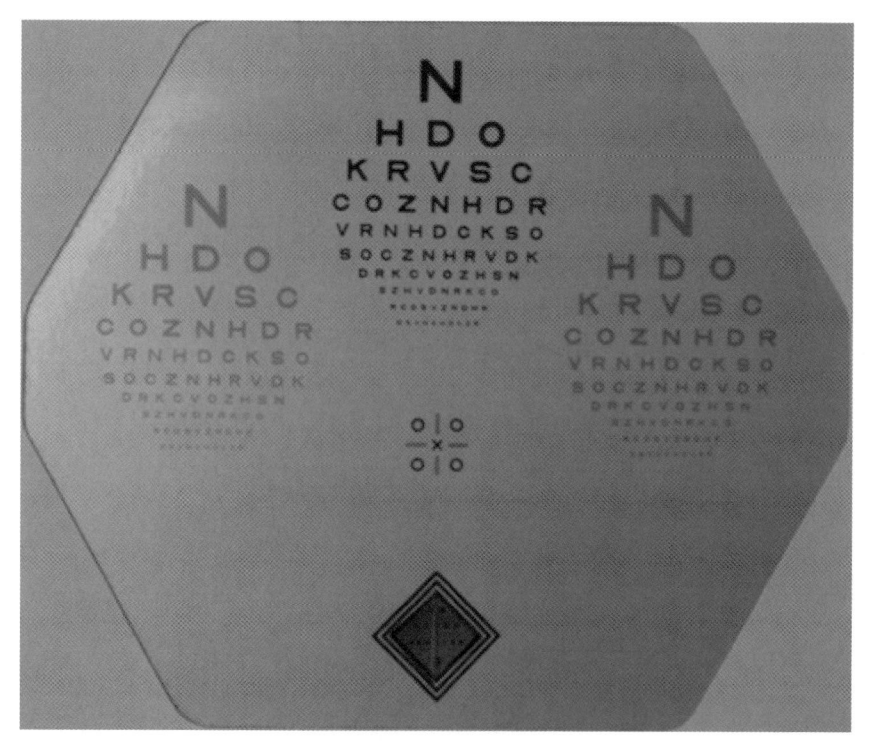

Figure 3: One side of the Borish Near Point Vectograph card. NOTE: This one was modified with extra Polaroids added to the small letter chart at the bottom to look for intermittent central suppression by the editor.

Let's take it for the hyperope 1+ 0.04(D) = AUH. Now let's take our 10D hyperope. 1 + 0.04(10) = 1 + 0.4=1.4. At 40cms = 2.50D x 1.4 = 3.50D. Now by using these units you can calculate much more accurately the accommodative demand for any patient with any given Rx in any kind of anisometropia or even with two different meridians. The point is what are we going to do about it if we find an uncorrected cylinder at near? You could make it in the segment – I get them that way once in awhile. The point is we have never demanded it. Why? Because, we've ignored it. Certainly when we start with a patient we all assume that our optics at least are right and that any problems that remain are other kinds of problems, and that's a legitimate assumption. But if we aren't doing our optics perfectly right, then we may sometimes be misleading ourselves in our other assumptions. That is the point I'm trying to make.

Do the cylinders change from far to near? Yes, they do. In one study, 10% showed a possible change and 14% in another study

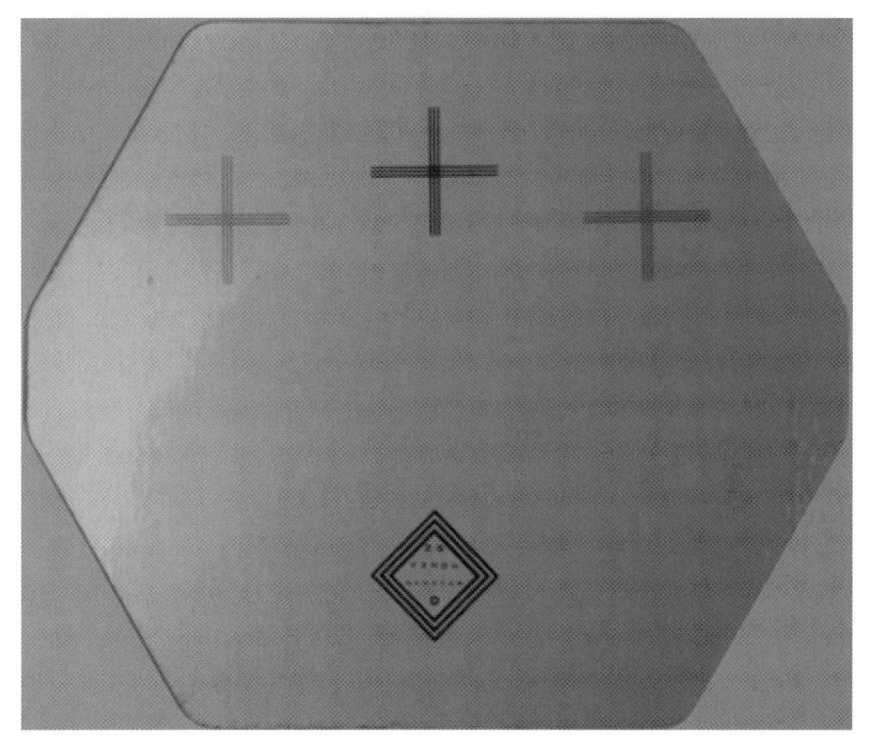

Figure 4: Here is the backside of the Borish Near Point Vectograph card. See text for description of the use of the card.

showed +/- 0.50D change in power monocularly from far to near, just through the lens effectivity changes and looking peripherally instead of centrally. Let me show you one of the great fallacies in our procedures. We work on the primary line of sight again. And what happens to the primary line of sight? When I converge this is what happens to my convergence and my line of sight; we end up with axis 90 in each eye. Now you give me the print to read and I drop it some 40 degrees downward and I converge down and watch my hands, and automatically whatever cylinder you've got in the distance has to be at the wrong axis for the reading.[3]

I have developed a near-point chart which has near-point Vectographs on both sides and it will fit on the reading rod or you can hold it in your hand. One side presents three cross cylinder test objects and a diamond with letters in it. The polarization is such that the average patient sees this with the right eye, the central cross cylinder target,

---
3. *Editors Note: Dr.Borish rotated his hands in opposite directions away from 90 degrees in each eye.*

the right one and the diamond, and this with the left eye, so that they see with both eyes, the central target binocularly, the right target monocularly, the left target monocularly and the diamond with both eyes. I use this for a comparison of binocular and monocular cross cylinder findings in comparison of accommodative activity This is not a test to substitute for a dissociated cross cylinder if you want to dissociate and take the cross cylinder

I say to the patient, "Is one set blacker than the other?" "Sure, the across ones are. The up and down are purple or blue or red," and time after time I get that. I say, "Are they more distinct one way than the other? Do they stand out better?" "Yes, the across ones stand out better." I say, "What about the right chart?" "Yes, the across ones." "What about the left chart?" "Yes, the across ones." "Tell me, do they change as I add these lenses," and I add plus. The patient may say, "Now wait a minute, the right one and the center one look alike but the left one's lines are still black, still more distinct crossways." A bell rings. Why? Is it possible that we have unequal accommodation? Did I miss the equalization at far? How much anisometropia is there? What happened and why is it different? And so I check the cross cylinders quickly, monocularly, binocularly and I make comparisons of the accommodative action of both eyes quickly.

Now I have them look at the diamond. What is the smallest print you can read in the diamond? That is 20/20 incidentally. The bottom line is 20/40, then comes 20/20, 20/25, 20/30. Why did we use the diamond? We used the diamond because, we must use and hold accommodation fixed. Suppose his acuity is so poor that he can't see any of the letters? He can see the three lines usually, the grid. If he says, "I can't see any letters," I'll say, "Can you see that pattern, the three-line pattern?" "Yes." "Keep that as clear as you can." Now here is what he sees and then I disassociate him, and here I've lined one over the other. You'll notice that the two diamonds are very simple to line up. Those top points give almost a very near alignment. I can have him look at the lower chart, the print in the lower chart because I don't know which way to play this game and so I always pick the lower one, and I say, "Look at the print in the lower chart and tell me without looking and while you keep that clear when do you think the upper one is right above it. With these Vernier arrow system pointers you'd be surprised how accurate they

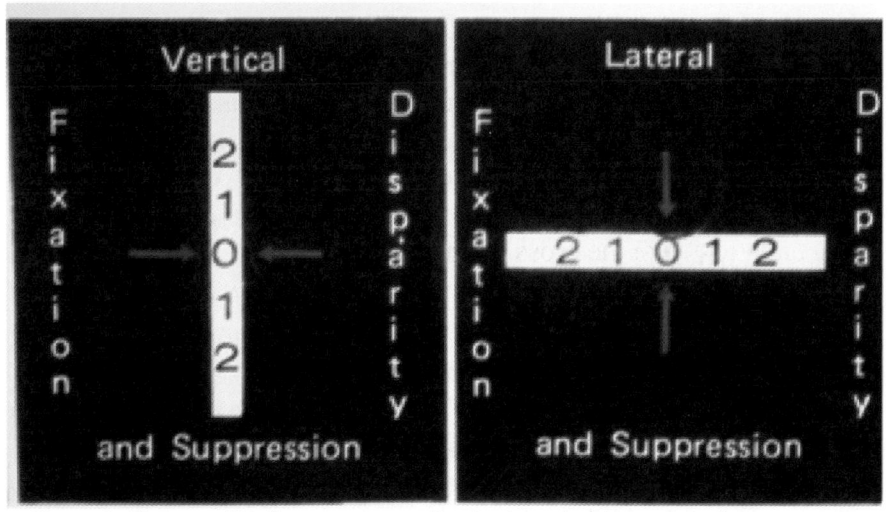

Figure 6: Close up of Mallett test targets. One horizontal and one vertical arrow are seen by each eye because of the Polaroids overlaid over the arrows.

can line that target up. And then I do it in reverse and we get the lateral and the vertical because they can line the other two points up. So I got the phorias, and now I turn the chart around and I got this target on the other side. Again I want you to look the same diamond as there was before. There are three charts going down to 20/20 and the disparity test. The problem here is this. I was told by Stereo Optical of Chicago that we could not make a 20/20 chart at near in Vectographs. And so we went into our own photographic laboratory and we made it, and after we showed it to them he said alright, and he made it, and so we did get 20/20 letters.

And so we're going down to the 20/20 line on all three charts, and again, just as with the front side, this is what the right eye sees. Both eyes see this. It's is a negative of it but you get the general idea of it. I ask the patient, "What is the smallest print you can read in the center chart?" I take his acuity at near with both eyes together. "What is the smallest print you can see in the right chart? In the left chart?" If he sees equal print in the two outside charts I'm happy but if he sees better in one chart than the other, again the bell rings. Why? I wonder if there might be a difference in accommodative effort, ability, equalization, a difference in my equalization or is something wrong at near.

Now if I want to take the amplitude of accommodation I can take it in any of the ways you may want to take it. You can take it by the adaptation of Sheard's method which is adding minus lenses, or you can take it by push-up, which is the Donders-Duane method. Both have advantages and disadvantages. On the Sheard method the common set of norms we use are applied and they shouldn't be because they were established by the Donders-Duane method. Whichever you use, if you know what you're using, it doesn't matter, but I take the amplitude with both eyes. I take it at the same time.

I want you to notice my language. I say to the patient, "I want you to watch the print in the diamond and as you watch it tell me if it becomes blurred. Or, tell me if the diamond doubles, or tell me if the diamond moves to either side," and that is the part we don't tell the patient. And so here's what happens to patients. You start to put a little stress on their convergence with base-out prism and they suppress their left eye and so the chart just moves along. It doesn't blur or double. Also I take prism base in instead of prism base out first. In the numbering scheme of the routine I wish that we could renumber the tests so that prism base in came ahead of prism base out in all the tests. Why? Many of you know the name Matthew Alpern,[4] who was probably one of the outstanding physicists in the world today and was an optometrist. Matthew, when he was a student at Northern Illinois College and I was teaching there, came to me right after graduation with his first experiment, a comparison of the reactions of prism base out following prism base in, and prism base in following prism base out. Comparison of vergences taken after phorias and phorias taken after vergences and how they affect each other and we take them all wrong. So now I teach our students not to take them the way we have them listed. The point is that all phorias ought to be taken before any ductions or any vergences. You can test that out. All base in should precede base out because base out will vastly affect base in comparison to the way base in affects base out. I always take my base in measurements first and then my base out measurements.

One other aspect we look at is the fixation disparity. This is not the best fixation disparity test in the world because to do this correctly we should have color differences. Mallett spent a great deal of time working out the exact size of the bar line and the color. He wants a green at near and a red at far and we have black and white and that's

---

4. Alpern M. *The eyes and vision.* In: *Handbook of Optics*, Section 12. McGraw Hill, 1978.

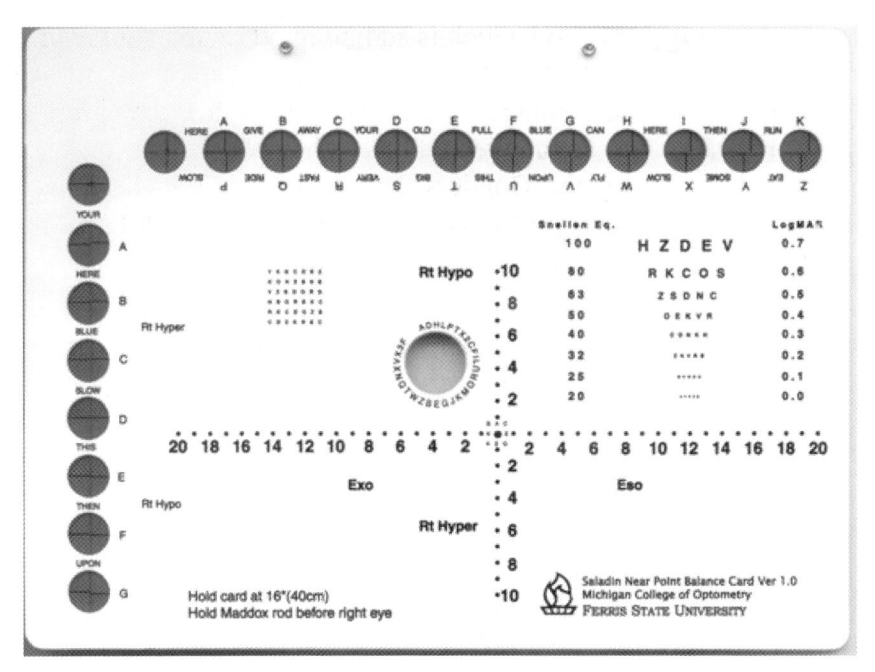

Figure 7: The Saladin card, which emerged much after the presentation of this paper.

not the best. Secondly, Mallett introduced another element that you must watch out for in all disparity tests, and that is that you must have strong peripheral fusion to take a true disparity otherwise what you're taking is some kind of irregular type of mixture of disparity and phorias. In the Mallett test there is a little circle with nonius[5] lines and a lot of print. In this test we get our fusional lock from the diamond from the central chart in addition to the cross and the little circles. This chart shows you a left hyper-disparity. You see, that little line is up even though everything is being fused. Disparity is a whole subject in its own and we are having a big talk at the Academy on disparity, and in addition we are working on entirely different angles of disparity. We are going back to Ogle. The Mallett test is not the best test. This is not the best test because it's based on the Mallett test The Ogle System seems to be much better and we are now developing Sheedy and Saladin who have developed a test target for disparity that introduces a wholly different new concept of

---

5. *Definition: a device for adjusting the accuracy of mathematical instruments, later superseded by the Vernier.*

how to test at near. That is added information on testing at near in a different vein.

One other thing, suppose I have a discrepancy in these targets, what can I do? I can take a cross cylinder, put an Rx in the trial frame, or leave it in the refractor. I can do it in the primary plane or the reading plane. If I did it in the reading plane I take the card down and give to the patient to hold it in the reading plane and I put the Rx in the trial frame. He looks at this card in a natural position and I take a hand-crossed cylinder out and I say, "Keep the left card as clear as you can but alternate between left and right, and while you're looking at the left one keep it as clear as you can, and looking at the right I'm going to blur the right one two different ways" and I take and recheck the cylinder with the hand-crossed cylinder at near. I then do the same with the left eye using the right eye to try to hold the accommodation. There's one thing about this card; it's my card and has my name on it. Vectographs are very expensive to make and this is a two-sided vectograph. The only thing about it is it needs a lot of light. Don't have your lamp way up here on the chair and have the card here. It won't be bright enough. The lamp must be close to it. I have enjoyed being with you these couple of days and I hope you have too. Thank you.